What Your Unborn Baby Wants You to Know

What Your Unborn Baby Wants You to Know

A Complete Guide to a Healthy Pregnancy

Boris Petrikovsky, M.D., Ph.D.,

Jessica Jacob, M.D.,

and Lisa Aiken, Ph.D.

A Perigee Book

The suggestions in this book are not intended to replace treatment by your physician. All questions and concerns regarding your health should be directed to your physician. The mention of specific products or brands in this book does not constitute an endorsement by either the authors or the publisher. The stories in this book are based on the experiences of actual people, but the names and circumstances have been altered to ensure confidentiality.

A Perigee Book
Published by The Berkley Publishing Group
A division of Penguin Putnam Inc.
375 Hudson Street
New York, New York 10014

Copyright © 2001 by Boris Petrikovsky, M.D., Ph.D., Jessica Jacob, M.D., and Lisa Aiken, Ph.D.
Book design by Tiffany Kukec
Cover design by Erika Fusari
Cover art by IT Itn'l/ estock/ picturequest
Figure 2 and figure 3 on pages 110 and 136 are used with the permission of Gene Care
All other illustrations are by Michael Gellatly

First edition: July 2001

Published simultaneously in Canada.

The Penguin Putnam Inc. World Wide Web site address is
www.penguinputnam.com

Library of Congress Cataloging-in-Publication Data

Petrikovsky, Boris M.
What your unborn baby wants you to know : a complete guide to a healthy pregnancy /
by Boris Petrikovsky, Jessica Jacob, and Lisa Aiken.
p.   cm.
Includes index.
ISBN 0-399-52682-X
1. Pregnancy—Popular works. 2. Childbirth—Popular works. 3. Prenatal care—Popular
works. I. Jacob, Jessica. II. Aiken, Lisa. III. Title.

RG525 .P437 2001
618.2'4—dc21   00-050127

Printed in the United States of America

10   9   8   7   6   5   4   3   2   1

*This book is dedicated to Muriel, who gave birth to five
wonderful children without benefit of this book.*
—BMP

*This book is also dedicated to my family, who has forever put up
with my unpredictable absences due to my profession.*
—JRJ

~ CONTENTS

PART III: *Labor and Delivery*

❧ ACKNOWLEDGMENTS

The authors wish to express their deep gratitude to Drs. James Macri, Terrence Hallahan, and David Krantz at the Neural Tube Defects Laboratory, John Rodis at the University of Connecticut Health Center, and Debra Lynn Day-Salvatore at the Robert Wood Johnson Medical School for contributing their valuable information to this book. We would also like to thank Dr. Anthony Vintzileos, professor of Obstetrics and Gynecology and Reproductive Sciences, for his valuable comments, and Drs. Susan Thalheim and Leon Zacharowicz for reviewing the manuscript.

W*hen a woman discovers that she is pregnant, she wants to know what* will happen to her and her baby during the next nine months. She wants to know how to protect and nurture her unborn child as much as possible. And while most pregnancies are trouble-free, women have individual concerns, applying to their particular circumstances, that they would like addressed. A significant number of new mothers are older, and that number is increasing all the time, so we have included information for the special concerns of pregnant women ages thirty-five and older.

Pregnant women want to know how their experiences or activities can affect their unborn children so they can take appropriate precautions. They want to know about everything from travel to hair dye and the effect it will have on their developing baby. They want to know how they can be reassured early in pregnancy that their babies are normal and what can be done to fix fetal problems before the baby is born.

This book is a resource that will help women safeguard the health of their unborn children. It tells mothers what they really want to know about their unborn babies in a readable, reassuring, and highly informative style, including information that has never before been available to laypeople. This is the only guide to pregnancy that was written by a world-renowned expert in the field of maternal-fetal medicine, using information that is well known only to those in this field, and by an extremely busy and experienced clinician who has seen it all.

Maternal-fetal medicine is a new branch of obstetrics which deals with high-risk mothers and their unborn babies. It is a specialty area that combines use of obstetrical ultrasound, measurements of the fetal environment, knowledge of genetics and infectious diseases, general medicine, and fetal surgery. Due to the rapid accumulation of knowledge in this area, even practicing obstetricians may not be aware of all of the research findings that may be relevant to their patients. Few patients could even imagine all the questions they need to ask in order to safeguard their baby's life or health.

Dr. Boris Petrikovsky has overseen the births of over ten thousand babies in his twenty-five years as an obstetrician. He is regarded as a doctor with few peers in the area of diagnostic fetal sonography and fetal development. He is a renowned researcher and clinician in fetal health and diagnosis. His knowledge comes from studying mothers and their unborn babies, and from working with other fetal researchers and surgeons on the cutting edge of this exciting specialty. This book was "tested" with patients, and their comments were incorporated in making this book user-friendly.

In the seventeen years during which Dr. Jessica Jacob has been delivering babies, she has taken care of thousands of pregnant women. She has calmed their fears, listened to their concerns, and explained to them what remained unclear and confusing. In the course of these busy years, she became acutely aware of what patients wanted and (even more important) needed to know to have a healthy baby. Much of the material in this guide is culled straight from the discussions that she engages in daily.

Besides enlightening the reader about the latest advances in maternal-fetal medicine, this book presents the material in a very accessible way. For example, rather than having chapters correspond to the weeks of pregnancy, and/or using a question and answer format, we discuss a series of related subjects that might impact the mother or fetus. This makes it easy for women to look up an area of concern in one section of our book instead of flipping through several chapters that discuss only bits and pieces. This should give the reader a more comprehensive and organized view of each topic, including how to know when problems warrant concern, and what can be done when action needs to be taken.

We organized this book according to normal circumstances that pregnant women encounter, medical problems that may arise, labor and delivery, and the postpartum period.

Finally, this book is unique in that it discusses topics that are relevant for today's woman, such as: What kinds of herbs are beneficial or harmful in pregnancy? What must a pregnant woman know about traveling to other countries? What special precautions should be taken when a woman is pregnant with twins or triplets? Will the fetus be normal if a woman gets pregnant while taking Prozac or other psychotropic medications? How can Lyme disease affect an unborn baby? What can be done to diagnose and treat fetal problems before the baby is born?

The majority of fetal problems can be prevented or treated when the expectant mother is well informed and she works with a competent and knowledgeable health care practitioner. While this book is not intended to replace a pregnant woman's health caretaker, and should not be used to self-treat medical or obstetrical problems, the information within can help pregnant women make educated choices about what to do and what questions to ask their health care practitioners during this very special time of their lives. No matter what the source of your information, always discuss any specific problems that arise during your pregnancy with your health caretaker.

What Your Unborn Baby Wants You to Know

PART I

Normal Pregnancy

CHAPTER ONE

Life Begins

*O*ne *of the most exciting moments in many women's lives is that* instant when they realize they are pregnant. Women come to this situation from many different vantage points. Some have dreamed of this moment from early childhood, and have spent years preparing themselves for motherhood. Others have spent half a lifetime without children before attempting to conceive. Still others are unpleasantly surprised at this unexpected turn of events, and may need time to get used to the idea that they will be mothers. Yet others have spent years and untold sums of money wishing and hoping for this moment to happen.

As the implications of this moment reach into every woman's heart, most will be overwhelmed by the thought that the most awesome, incredible event in the entire universe is happening to them. They have within them a work in progress that will end with their creation of a tiny human being.

The baby inside them becomes a main focus of their thoughts and feelings over the next nine months. Expectant mothers wonder, "How big is my baby now? What position is it in? What does it look like? What sex is it? Will eating my favorite junk foods hurt it? What is the baby doing now? Can he hear me when I speak to him?" As the woman's body changes and she feels her baby move, she bonds more and more with the tiny person developing within her.

In order to better appreciate the amazing changes that mother and baby go through during their nine-month journey together, we will describe what a woman's reproductive system looks like, how it works, and what changes it goes through during pregnancy.

The Uterus

The womb, or uterus, is a muscular organ that looks like an upside-down pear sitting in the middle of a woman's pelvis. Filmy tissue connects it to the bladder, which sits in front of it. This positioning explains why the enlarged uterus presses down on the bladder as pregnancy progresses, making women need to urinate often.

When women are not pregnant, the uterus is the size of a fist, with the front and back walls collapsed almost against each other. A hollow, thin-walled fallopian tube attaches each side of the uterus to an ovary (see fig. 1). When ectopic pregnancies (those outside of the uterus) occur, they are usually in one of these flimsy fallopian tubes.

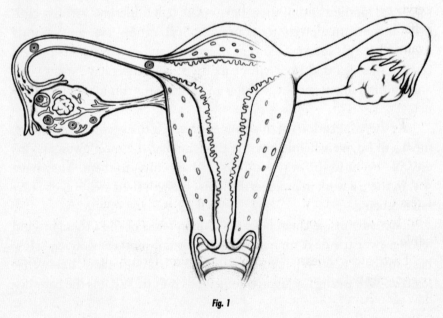

Fig. 1

The uterus is lined with a tissue called endometrium. It builds up every month in preparation for nourishing an embryo, and it continues to develop if a pregnancy occurs. Alternatively, it degrades and sheds, causing menstruation, if it is not used.

The endometrium "knows" what to do because it gets signals from two female hormones called estrogen and progesterone. The ovaries make these hormones when women are not pregnant, as well as during the first eleven weeks of pregnancy.

The Cervix

The neck of the uterus, or cervix, is long, cylindrical, and firm, and sits at the top of the vagina. (This is what the practitioner swabs when a Pap smear is done.) The cervix feels like the tip of one's nose because it is mostly fibrous tissue and collagen. Collagen makes the tip of the nose and the ears hard, and also keeps the cervix hard enough to maintain a baby in the uterus for nine months. When the cervix is weak, the baby can actually drop from the uterus.

Normally, the cervix "ripens" at the end of pregnancy, and much of the collagen breaks down and is replaced by water. This makes the cervix soft and pliable. It then starts opening up (dilating) and thinning (effacing) when there are uterine contractions and a baby's head presses against it.

The Ovaries

The ovaries are almond-shaped organs on either side of the uterus. Each month, one part of the brain tells the pituitary gland in another part of the brain to signal one ovary to release an egg (ovulate). Because the brain's messages are affected by one's emotional state, it is easy for stress to play havoc with the menstrual cycle. This is also why women who live or work together may even get synchronized periods after a while.

Each ovary releases an egg every other month. If a woman has twenty-eight-day menstrual cycles, ovulation usually occurs thirteen days after her period started, or fourteen days before the next period begins. The egg then disintegrates twelve to twenty-four hours later, unless it is fertilized by a sperm during this time. If a couple wants to get pregnant, they should have intercourse every other day during the middle of the woman's cycle. Because sperm live for at least forty-eight hours outside of the man's body, that frequency of sex will keep live sperm in the fallopian tube awaiting the egg's arrival. If a woman's periods are very irregular or infrequent and she has difficulty getting pregnant, she should consult her practitioner about ways to improve her chances of conceiving.

When a woman's ovary releases an egg every month, the part of the ovary from which the egg came, the corpus luteum (literally, "yellow body") makes estrogen and progesterone. This extra progesterone tells the uterine lining to build up. About eleven days after ovulation, the corpus luteum starts to break down if pregnancy hasn't occurred. The reduction in hormones that the corpus luteum had been making signals the endometrium to disintegrate, and the woman gets her period.

If pregnancy does occur, the woman's body makes human chorionic gonadatropin (HCG), which signals the endometrium not to break down, and the corpus luteum continues to make enough estrogen and progesterone to maintain the pregnancy until about eleven weeks. From then on until the end of the pregnancy, the placenta makes the necessary pregnancy hormones.

Placenta

The placenta, or "afterbirth," is an amazing organ that weighs about one and a half pounds. It brings nutrients and oxygen to the baby and takes away its waste. It also makes the hormones that are critical to pregnancy. Huge veins and arteries bring enormous amounts of blood through the placenta, which is why any disease that ages or harms the blood vessels could also damage the placenta and interfere with the baby getting what it needs. High blood pressure, diabetes, lupus, and even "old age" can make a woman high risk for maintaining a pregnancy.

Umbilical Cord

The baby is connected to the placenta by the umbilical cord, which is a soft, pliable, and Jell-O–like hose that contains two arteries and a vein in a gel-like substance. The two arteries remove waste products from the baby, and the vein brings the baby oxygen-rich blood. Mothers often worry about kinking or constricting the baby's umbilical cord, but the blood vessels are so full of blood that they are too rigid to kink; in addition, the gel prevents kinking.

The umbilical cord normally floats in cushioning amniotic fluid (basically urine from the fetus) unless the placenta is not doing its job. When the placenta is healthy, the baby gets enough fluid to urinate well and create a normal amount of amniotic fluid. That, in turn, cushions the umbilical cord.

Although most women have heard about them, umbilical cord catastrophes are very rare. While 25–33 percent of babies are born with an umbilical cord around their necks, it is extremely unusual for a baby to be born dead because it was strangled by its cord. As long as a fetus's activity level is normal, the overwhelming likelihood is that the baby will be okay.

Showing

Most women get excited about "showing." That happens when the baby and the amniotic fluid inside the uterus push against the uterine walls, making them expand. The uterus usually grows as the baby does, with two exceptions: Women with fibroids (benign tumors of the uterus) may have growths that get larger as the pregnancy progresses, making it look as if the baby is larger than it actually is. Women who are polyhydramniotic have too much amniotic fluid and also appear larger.

How "big" a woman is during pregnancy depends upon many factors: how well toned her abdominal muscles are, whether she has already had a baby, the position of the baby, how tall she is (taller women tend not to show as much), how big the baby is, and so on. Some women will wear maternity clothes toward the end of their first trimester, while others can disguise their pregnancy until twenty-eight weeks. Women who already have a child generally show earlier in subsequent pregnancies than they did the first time around.

Practitioners can usually tell how big the baby is by feeling where the top of the uterus (fundus) is. Some practitioners are more comfortable using a tape measure to determine fundal height, but a seasoned practitioner can usually tell how big the baby is by gently feeling with the hands.

How the Baby Is Born

For most women, after thirty-seven to forty-two weeks of pregnancy, the body sends out a hormone called oxytocin, which causes the walls of the uterus to contract. This is the beginning of labor. These contractions pull at the top of the cervix, making it thin and open up. Meanwhile, the baby's head pushes down on the cervix during contractions, further opening the cervix. This opening and thinning of the cervix causes a mucus plug that seals off the cervix to be dislodged. Some blood vessels normally break and cause light bleeding when the plug moves.

The latent, or early phase of labor occurs when the cervix is less than four centimeters dilated and contractions are relatively mild. When women say their labor lasted one or two days, they are referring to this stage of labor. Some women have latent labor for a few hours, others have it for as much as a few days—everyone is different. If this part of labor goes well, it makes the active, more painful part of labor much easier.

The active phase of labor starts when the woman's cervix is about four centimeters dilated and continues until the baby is born. If the labor doesn't progress well, the practitioner may give the woman some Pitocin (the commercially prepared form of oxytocin) through an intravenous line in order to speed things up. The practitioner also determines if progress is delayed because the baby is too big to fit through the mother's pelvis or is in a bad position for a vaginal birth.

When the woman's cervix is ten centimeters dilated, stage one labor ends and stage two labor begins. Stage two starts when the woman begins pushing and it ends with the birth of the baby. Stage three is the time between the birth of the baby and the expulsion of the placenta. When a woman has a cesarean section, the baby can be removed in about a minute. It can take anywhere from a minute to a half hour during a vaginal delivery.

The six weeks after the placenta is expelled is called the postpartum. During that time, the uterus gradually returns to normal and the woman adjusts to having a new baby.

Weeks One to Four

During the nine months of pregnancy, profound changes happen to the baby.

Conception occurs when a man's sperm penetrates the membrane of an egg released by the woman's ovary into her fallopian tube. The egg is now fertilized and it contains bits of information from both the mother's and the father's genes in the form of twenty-three chromosomes that each parent contributes. The first twenty-two pairs of chromosomes determine the baby's genetic potentials. Will it have blue or brown eyes? Will it be tall or short? Will it have its mother's ear for music or its father's athletic build? Every child inherits a unique combination of his parents' genes, except for identical twins, who share the same genes.

The twenty-third chromosome determines the baby's sex. Women contribute an X chromosome to every child, while fathers determine the baby's sex by contributing either an X or a Y chromosome. Girls have two X chromosomes, one contributed by each parent, while boys have an X from the mother and a Y from the father.

The chromosomes tell the fertilized egg, a single cell, to grow and divide into a many-celled structure called a zygote, which travels from the fallopian tube into the uterus during a three-day journey. It then hovers freely for another three days in the uterus, where it is nourished by secretions from glands there. By the end of the first week after conception, this ball burrows into the lining of the uterus. It usually does this near the top of the back wall of the uterus. This is where the placenta tends to be when the woman delivers. Occasionally, implantation can occur low in the uterus, close to, or even covering, the cervix, in a condition called placenta previa. (See page 190.)

When implantation occurs, it breaks up some blood vessels, sometimes causing painless, light vaginal spotting. This is called implantation bleeding. Now called a blastocyst, the ball of cells gets its oxygen and nutrition directly from the mother's uterine lining.

The uterus has been preparing for its new arrival by thickening and enriching its blood supply with the help of progesterone made by the ovary. Soon after the blastocyst enters the uterus, the cells divide into two layers: The outer layer eventually forms what will be a placenta, and the inner part becomes an embryo.

The outer part makes a critical hormone called human chorionic gonadatropin (HCG). HCG signals the ovary not to stop making estrogen and progesterone. Without HCG, the ovary would stop making progesterone and the woman would shed the uterine lining through menstruation. With HCG, the ovary makes lots of progesterone until the placenta takes over this function around week eleven. Progesterone helps the uterine lining get thicker and thicker as the pregnancy advances. Not only is HCG critical for the success of the pregnancy, it affords us a handy way of knowing if a woman is pregnant or not. By a few days before a newly pregnant woman expects her period, her body is making enough HCG to be detected on a blood test. By the time she expects her period, her urine will have enough HCG in it to be detected by a home pregnancy test.

When a woman gets a positive pregnancy test, she first becomes aware that a new life is growing inside her. By that time, a lot has already happened.

How the Baby Grows

Although a woman may not look pregnant, her growing baby has already gone through some amazing changes by the time her pregnancy is confirmed. Research studies tell us that all of the cells in the preliminary ball of cells could become almost anything. Then, a signal goes out among them so that each cell is cued by the others to develop a certain way. The result is that a miniature human being develops. If anything disturbs the timing or location of these signals, the ultimate baby that is in the making can be affected. This is the time when the baby's organs start developing rapidly, and they are vulnerable to toxins until they are completed during the next few weeks. This is when it is most important to stay away from toxins and medications that might cause birth defects.

At the start of the third week after conception, blood vessels start forming, and a rudimentary circulatory system starts to work. The embryonic blood cells get nutrients and oxygen from, and get rid of waste products through, the mother's blood. By the end of the third week the embryo's heart has developed four chambers (two atria and two ventricles) and started beating. This is the first of the baby's organ systems to function. Although we can't hear the heart beating, we can see a faint but definite pulsation on specialized ultrasound. (Ultrasound is another name for sonogram.)

The forerunner of the spinal cord, called the neural tube, also develops during this same time, as do the spaces in the embryo that eventually give rise to body cavities.

Around this time the chorionic villi also start to form. These are fingerlike projections that securely attach the embryo to the lining of the uterus. The embryo's blood first flows across these villi, which eventually become the placenta. The baby-in-making requires enough maternal blood bathing these villi. If the mother has certain diseases, such as high blood pressure or diabetes, or if she smokes heavily, this interferes with blood flow and can seriously impair the baby's growth and development.

Weeks Five to Eight

These are critical weeks of development, as all of the baby's major structures develop at this time (except for the cardiovascular system, which is already up and running). The embryo initially looks like it has a curved tail, but the tail disappears at the end of this time. The embryo also develops limb buds, which will become arms and legs.

By the end of the fourth week after conception, the baby is a fifth of an inch long. Its respiratory system is starting to form, as are its esophagus, stomach, liver, and pancreas.

During the fifth week after conception, the head grows rapidly, the face starts to form, and kidneys start to develop. Embryos start to move now.

During the sixth week after conception, the paddle-shaped arms start to develop elbows and hands, and the eyes can now be seen clearly.

During the seventh week, the hands get notches, which will later differentiate into fingers. The intestines grow so quickly that the baby's tiny abdomen can't hold them, and they are forced to travel into the umbilical cord for a short time. Arm bones start to form by the end of this week.

During the eighth week after conception, one can see webbed fingers and toes, and bones that have started forming in the legs. The eyelids that start forming will stay closed until the seventh month. The baby now has ears as well. The baby is already moving purposefully although the mother can't feel it yet.

Weeks Nine to Twelve

The baby's body elongates now, as calcium gets deposited throughout its skeleton.

The thyroid and pancreas are formed during the tenth week, and the pancreas starts making insulin a week later. The baby can now suck his fingers and make his hand into a fist. It also moves about and urinates in the amniotic fluid. This fluid consists of water, a few nutrients, and some skin cells shed by the baby. Amniotic fluid is initially made by the cells lining the pregnancy sac; eventually, it consists mostly of the baby's urine. When women have a procedure called amniocentesis, the doctor withdraws some of the baby's cells in this fluid to see if the baby's chromosomes are normal. This fluid contains cells that the fetus sheds; these can be grown in a lab and then studied under a microscope.

The intestines that developed outside the baby's body migrate back into the abdomen between weeks eleven and twelve. Rarely, they stay in the umbilical cord until birth, in which case the problem is readily remedied with surgery. This condition is also one reason why practitioners try not to clamp the umbilical cord too close to the abdomen when a baby is born.

By the end of this time, the baby has fingernails and swallows amniotic fluid. Vocal cords, lips, and a nose are developing. By the twelfth week, external genitalia are more identifiable, although they can't be definitively seen until fourteen weeks. The baby now weighs about one-half ounce and is a little over two inches long. Most women are not yet wearing maternity clothes, but most of the baby's organs and tissues are already formed.

Weeks Thirteen to Sixteen

Babies grow rapidly at this time. By thirteen weeks, fetal researchers can see babies breathe, suck, hiccup, and swallow amniotic fluid, even though the baby weighs only one ounce! Babies now have all of the major organs, and they start gaining weight. At the same time, mothers start making more blood in order to nourish the growing fetus.

The fetal bones are all calcified now, making them easy to see on ultrasound. Until now, the eyes have been sitting on either side of the head, much like a bird's. At this point, they face forward, giving the baby a much more human appearance.

The ovaries and testes also form around this time. By fifteen weeks, the average baby weighs three to four ounces and measures about four inches long. Women who want prenatal testing can get an alpha-fetoprotein (AFP) blood test or amniocentesis done around this time.

Weeks Seventeen to Twenty

Fetal movements can be felt reliably by the mother at some time during this three-week period because the baby's bones are harder and his muscles are stronger. These movements are important in helping the baby develop its muscles as well as its brain. If the baby stayed still in the uterus for a long time (which it doesn't), it would not develop correctly.

The baby's skin is very thin and has no fat under it, so it makes a perfect moisturizer called vernix. This creamy, greasy, protective layer of white lotion envelops it, preventing the skin from "pruning up" and ripping during its prolonged amniotic bath. (It is made by the same sebaceous glands that produce the oil and acne that are the bane of adolescents.)

The vernix starts to disappear close to the time of delivery. Babies who are born with a thick coat of vernix were probably born before their due date.

The baby now has all of his hair follicles. He has hair on his head and eyebrows, with a fine, downy hair called lanugo on the rest of his body. (Lanugo disappears close to term.) A female fetus already has ovaries and eggs, with a uterus and vagina forming by eighteen weeks. The baby's teeth start forming, although they won't push through the gums until the baby is about six months old.

The baby's brain develops rapidly now, especially the frontal lobe—the center of intelligence.

The fetus may be able to hear sounds now.

The placenta is well developed, and there are about four to six ounces of amniotic fluid. The baby now weighs about eleven ounces and is about six inches long.

The baby's major organ and skeletal systems, as well as the spine, can be clearly seen on ultrasound (often for the first time) now. If need be, the fetal heart can also be examined by ultrasound. Many pregnant women are sent for ultrasounds at this time.

Weeks Twenty-one to Twenty-four

The fetus now looks like a skinny, wrinkled, red baby. Loud, sudden noises will cause him to startle, even blink, and his heart rate may momentarily quicken. He may be familiarizing himself with sounds that he hears often. Many mothers say their babies move more, and sometimes rhythmically, in response to music. This is known as fetal dancing. Fetuses begin to recognize their mother's voice and, according to some researchers, are calmed by it. Eyelids may be open by now.

The baby is about eight inches long and weighs a little more than a pound.

By twenty-four weeks, the baby has distinct footprints and fingerprints. When he is born, the hospital will take footprints because the baby's hands will stay clenched for some time after birth.

At this time the baby starts making small amounts of surfactant, an

important component of the lung. When there is more of it, it will prevent collapse of the little air pockets that make up the lungs. Babies
born at this time rarely live because their lungs are too immature.

Weeks Twenty-five to Twenty-nine

At this stage, more babies are able to live outside the uterus. Their
brains can control rhythmic breathing movements and body temperature, and they start to fill out with fat.

By twenty-six weeks, the baby's eyes are always open, and the spleen
takes over the making of blood cells from the liver.

By twenty-eight weeks, the bone marrow starts making blood cells
and continues to do so for the rest of the baby's life.

Calcium is stored and the baby's bones harden.

Most babies now move into the fetal position—head down, rump
up, with legs bent at the knees and against the face—in preparation for
birth.

Weeks Thirty to Thirty-five

The baby now makes breathing motions (real breathing can't occur
until he is in contact with air) and hiccups. He kicks strongly and often
sticks a recognizable fist, elbow, or heel against the mother's abdomen.

He now stores iron and other minerals. (The iron stored before birth
will be used by the baby during the first six months of life.) The lanugo
has disappeared, the baby is getting plumper, and his pupils are respond-
ing to light.

The baby is now almost a foot long and weighs about three and a
half pounds. He is cushioned by about two pints of amniotic fluid.

Weeks Thirty-six to Forty

Babies gain about a half pound every week until they weigh about
seven and a half pounds at forty weeks. The baby may seem to be less active, although he continues to move almost every hour. The number of

movements should not change, although their force may seem feebler. The lungs are now mature, the head is (hopefully) positioned against the cervix, and he's ready to be born! Babies can safely be born at any time during this period.

Mothers often want to know how big their babies are at various points in the pregnancy. The accompanying table shows average fetal weights and lengths during the last four months of pregnancy. The specifics for your baby can be estimated by prenatal ultrasound.

Approximate Fetal Weights and Lengths for the Last Sixteen Weeks of Pregnancy

NUMBER OF WEEKS	WEIGHT	LENGTH IN INCHES
25	1 lb. 12 oz.	14.0
26	2 lb.	14.4
27	2 lb. 3 oz.	15.2
28	2 lb. 7 oz.	16.0
29	2 lb. 10 oz.	16.4
30	2 lb. 15 oz.	16.8
31	3 lb. 2 oz.	17.4
32	3 lb. 9 oz.	18.0
33	4 lb.	18.4
34	4 lb. 13 oz.	18.8
35	5 lb. 5 oz.	19.2
36	6 lb. 2 oz	19.6
37	6 lb. 8 oz.	19.8
38	6 lb. 10 oz.	20.0
39	7 lb. 4 oz.	20.2
40	7 lb. 15 oz.	20.4

Babies' weights normally vary a great deal once they reach the twenty-eighth week. Before then, their weights are pretty uniform, making ultrasounds more accurate in dating a pregnancy.

When Am I Due?

Health professionals date a pregnancy from a woman's last menstrual period (LMP), not from the time the egg actually got fertilized. Even if we know exactly when conception occurred, it is impossible to predict the exact date a baby will be born because each baby needs a different amount of time to develop in the uterus.

A woman's due date, also known as the estimated date of confinement (EDC), is the day the baby is expected to arrive. It is assumed that the baby will be born forty weeks from the woman's last menstrual period, or 267 days from the time the baby was actually conceived, even though this assumption is accurate only 6 percent of the time.

The actual calculation of a due date can be done in two ways:

• Count forty weeks from the start of the last menstrual period.

• Use Nagle's rule: Add seven days to the first day of the last menstrual period, then subtract three months. If a woman's last period started on June 14, add seven to get June 21, then subtract three months to get a due date of March 21.

However, these calculations are based on the often incorrect assumption that every woman has a twenty-eight-day cycle in which conception occurred on day fourteen. If your cycle is longer or shorter than twenty-eight days your due date will vary accordingly.

Adding to the confusion is the fact that health practitioners use weeks to determine the length of the pregnancy and women think of their pregnancies in terms of months. So if you want to know what month you are in, a rough way of figuring it out is to subtract from your due date. If it is March 21, you will be seven months pregnant on January 22. Your practitioner will consider you to be thirty-three weeks pregnant.

Myths

Being pregnant is full of mysteries and miracles, and wives' tales about having babies abound. Here are some that have no validity:

1. *If the baby has a fast heart rate it's a girl; if it's slow, it's a boy.*

2. *If the mother's belly is pointy, and her face is thin and pointy, it's a boy. If the mother's belly is round and her face is plumping out, it's a girl.*

3. *One can choose the baby's sex by varying the frequency of intercourse and the acidity of the woman's vagina.* Even though this received front-page coverage in *Life* magazine a couple of decades ago, controlled studies showed that these techniques are worthless.

4. *A baby with a full head of hair will cause the mother to get heartburn.*

5. *If a pregnant woman reaches her hands high above her head, such as when getting an item out of a cupboard, it may cause the umbilical cord to loop around the baby's neck.*

6. *Having a pelvic exam during the first trimester may cause a miscarriage.* Actually, although miscarriages are common during the first trimester, pelvic exams do not cause them.

7. *Walking or eating lobsters (!) close to the due date will cause a woman to go into labor.* Neither walking nor eating specific foods hastens labor.

8. *A full moon makes the bag of waters break and sends women into labor.*

9. *The baby should move less often toward the end of pregnancy because there is less room in the uterus.* This myth is dangerous. Babies should move well until the time of delivery. If a baby starts moving less close to the due date, it may be because there is too little amniotic fluid, in which case the baby will need to be delivered soon. If this happens, a woman should call her practitioner.

One "myth" that may be true is that having sex close to term will bring on labor—because semen contains prostaglandins, which ripen the cervix.

CHAPTER TWO

The First Prenatal Visit

*F*or many women, *the first sign of pregnancy is missing their period. If* they use a home pregnancy kit and it is positive, they should see their obstetrical caretaker around the time they are seven weeks pregnant. That is the same time as five weeks after they conceived. This is early enough for the woman to discuss important matters about the pregnancy with the health professional, but not so early that it's unclear if the pregnancy is likely to proceed.

Hopefully, the woman will have been taking .4 milligrams of folic acid every day before getting pregnant, in order to reduce the baby's chance of having birth defects. If she is having a high-risk pregnancy, she should take .8 milligrams. She should also have had her immunity to rubella (German measles) tested before getting pregnant. Women who once had rubella are immune for life, but women who were vaccinated may not be. Women who are no longer immune should be vaccinated before getting pregnant. The rubella vaccine should not be given during pregnancy.

At the first prenatal visit, and every subsequent one, the woman either brings a urine sample from the first time she urinates in the morning, or provides a urine specimen at the practitioner's office. The urine will be dipped with a strip of paper that has squares on it that change color when immersed in different chemicals. The caretaker looks at the squares for signs of infection. If the results seem suggestive, the woman will be asked to give a "clean catch" (midstream) urine specimen that is cultured for bacteria.

Pregnant women can have urinary tract infections with or without symptoms. These infections can lead to kidney infections, kidney stones, or preterm labor if left untreated.

Next, the urine is checked for sugar. Some pregnant women who are not diabetic have kidneys that leak sugar into the urine, but sugar in the urine suggests possible diabetes. If diabetic testing is normal, the spilling of sugar into the urine is ignored. If diabetes is present, it must be treated.

Finally, the urine is checked for protein to see if there is kidney disease. Most often, protein in the urine is due to some vaginal discharge that accidentally got into the urine specimen. If need be, a blood test can check blood urea nitrogen (BUN) and creatinine. If it is normal, the kidneys are functioning.

When there is a lot of protein in the urine toward the end of pregnancy, accompanied by swollen hands, face, and legs, and high blood pressure, it suggests toxemia. (See page 156 for more on toxemia.)

Medical History

Your practitioner will need information about your medical history at your first prenatal visit. It is important that you be able to tell your caretaker the following:

- *Have you ever had high blood pressure?* High blood pressure before pregnancy automatically makes a woman "high risk" because she may have abnormal blood vessels that will not nourish a placenta properly. Such women also have a much greater chance of getting toxemia toward the end of pregnancy, and a slightly higher chance that the placenta will separate from the uterine wall.

    Some women think they may have blood pressure that is too low, but that is almost never true. When such women feel faint, it is usually caused by long periods of standing or by getting up very quickly. Less commonly, low blood sugar, often due to not eating adequately, can also cause faintness.

- *Do you have heart disease?* Pregnancy stresses the heart in ways that most young, healthy women can handle, but those with some pre-existing heart conditions may not. Such women may need to be watched closely by a high-risk obstetrician and a cardiologist, who may recommend a cesarean section to avoid the stress of labor and delivery.

  If the condition of a woman's heart valves requires her to take antibiotics before getting dental treatment, she may need to take the same before she delivers. She should ask her cardiologist or internist about this and let her obstetrician know if any medications will be needed.

- *Do you have asthma?* Asthmatics must take their medication during pregnancy in order to ensure that the baby gets enough oxygen. If the mother doesn't get enough oxygen, the baby will suffer far more than it might from the medications themselves. It is fine for asthmatic women to take steroids when they need them at any time during pregnancy.

- *Do you have any kidney problems?* Women with kidney disease are more likely to have toxemia and babies that don't grow enough. These mothers are watched closely during pregnancy, and the baby's growth is monitored via ultrasound. Women who have had kidney transplants are often delivered early in order to avoid complications.

- *Do you have diabetes?* Diabetes must be well controlled during pregnancy. Diabetic women are advised to see their doctors before getting pregnant to try to ensure that conception occurs under the best possible circumstances. Diabetics are watched closely during pregnancy because of their greater risk of complications. They may get sonograms and non-stress tests as early as twenty-eight weeks.

- *Do you have migraine headaches?* The newer "miracle" drugs like Imitrex and Zomig can absolutely not be taken during pregnancy, and anti-inflammatory drugs like Motrin are discouraged. Extra-strength Tylenol is the best alternative, although Fioricet may be used judiciously when necessary.

• *Do you have a neurological condition?* Women with multiple sclerosis should consult their neurologist before getting pregnant. How multiple sclerosis will affect, or be affected by, a pregnancy is unpredictable.

• *Paraplegic and quadriplegic* women who have no sensation in their pelvic areas will not be able to feel uterine contractions or labor. They must be monitored closely throughout pregnancy and often have labor induced to make sure that they are in a safe place when they deliver.

• *Have you had scoliosis or back surgery?* Some back problems, such as some forms of severe scoliosis or having a Harrington rod, may make epidural administration almost impossible during labor and delivery. Women with these conditions can get other forms of anesthesia if they need it for pain relief, for a forceps delivery or cesarean section. Tell your caretaker if you have had scoliosis. If it is mild, many anesthesiologists can still give you a good epidural. Your caretaker may want to see medical and surgical records from orthopedists or neurosurgeons who treated you.

• *Do you have bad hip problems?* If so, tell your caretaker because it may affect the position in which you can deliver. If you have an epidural, your hip joint can be overstretched during labor and delivery without your realizing it until after the anesthesia has worn off.

• *Have you ever had a sexually transmitted disease?* If you have had herpes, there is a small chance that an outbreak could occur during delivery. That would require a cesarean section so the baby will not be exposed as he is delivered. Chlamydia can damage the Fallopian tubes and may increase a woman's chance of having an ectopic pregnancy.

• *Do you smoke cigarettes?* If so, your baby may not grow well, and your caretaker will have to monitor your baby's development closely.

- *Do you use illicit drugs or alcohol?* If so, your baby may be born addicted and will have to be watched in the nursery for symptoms of withdrawal. He may also be small or have birth defects, especially of the heart or brain.

- *Do you take any prescribed or over-the-counter medications?* Your caretaker needs to know about any medications that you take, because some of these may affect the fetus. Some should not be used at all during pregnancy; others may be safe; while still others may be used along with careful monitoring of the baby.

- *Do you have any allergies?* Women should be able to list all medications to which they have had definite allergic reactions, as well as those they avoid because a close relative is allergic. They should also tell their caretaker about side effects of medications, such as yeast infections with penicillin, or nausea with erythromycin. The latter are not allergies, but are drug reactions.

  Latex allergies have become prevalent of late, and a sensitized woman may have an extreme allergic reaction called anaphylaxis if she is examined with latex gloves during labor. That might cause her to stop breathing and require a ventilator temporarily until the allergic reaction ends.

- *Have any of your, or your partner's, relatives had birth defects, mental retardation, cystic fibrosis, heart defects, or neural tube defects?* Since some of these are inherited, knowing one's family history can help the caretaker know which problems to watch for.

  If you have other children with birth defects or developmental problems, tell your practitioner. Most anomalies do not recur, but a few do. If a previous child had spina bifida or a heart defect, there is a 3–5 percent chance that another baby will, too. If a sibling is autistic, there is up to a 7 percent chance that another boy will have it, and far less likelihood for girls.

  Fragile X is the most common inheritable form of mental retardation and developmental delay in American males. If a prior son was born with developmental delays, or if a male relative is mentally retarded, fetuses can be tested for fragile X if it is specifically requested when an amniocentesis is done.

- *What are your, and your partner's, ethnic backgrounds?* Different diseases affect different ethnic groups, and your caretaker may want to do genetic testing for those that are relevant to your baby. African-Americans should be tested for the sickle-cell anemia trait, Italians for thalessemia, whites for cystic fibrosis, and Ashkenazic Jews for Tay-Sachs, Canavan's, cystic fibrosis, and Gaucher's.

- *What have your prior pregnancies and deliveries been like?* Some obstetrical problems tend to repeat themselves. If prior births have been spontaneous vaginal deliveries with no complications, chances are excellent that this pattern will repeat itself. If one or more prior deliveries were done by cesarean section, the doctor should discuss the merits and drawbacks of having another cesarean section versus trying to deliver vaginally. Breech babies and fetal distress may both necessitate cesarean section for one baby, but do not tend to recur with subsequent babies. That is not the case when a cesarean section was done because the baby could not come out.

  If prior vaginal deliveries occurred so quickly that a woman barely made it to the hospital, or if there was early effacement and opening of the cervix, some practitioners will recommend inducing labor near term the next time.

  When prior births were premature because of early labor, women will be closely watched and advised to rest.

  If prematurity was due to a weak cervix, with silent opening and thinning of the cervix, stitching up the cervix after eleven weeks is advised. This is after most miscarriages would have occurred, but before the cervix has had a chance to thin out and malfunction.

  If a prior baby was small, the current pregnancy will be watched closely for the same. If a prior baby was very large, early maternal testing for diabetes will be done. The woman may also be advised to stay home and rest as much as possible.

If a woman had a few early miscarriages, she should be tested for blood factors that can attack the baby. She will also be seen more often than usual so that the caretaker can see if the pregnancy is proceeding, as well as to give the mother extra emotional support.

If a woman had early, severe toxemia or a blood clot in a previous pregnancy, she should get a certain blood test called an anticardiolipin antibody profile.

Always tell your practitioner about any bleeding problems you have had during prior pregnancies, surgeries or other medical/dental procedures, or if anyone in your family has bleeding problems such as von Willebrand's disease. If so, your blood clotting ability should be tested with a simple blood test. If you have a clotting disorder, a hematologist can determine what is missing so that it, and appropriate medications, can be supplied when you deliver.

The Physical Exam

After taking your medical and obstetrical history, your practitioner will measure your blood pressure. This will give a basis for comparing later blood pressures. Normally, a blood pressure of 130/85 is considered borderline, while 130+/90 or higher is considered high. If a woman's first blood pressure measures only 90/60 (on the low side), rather than in the normal range of 110/60 to 125/85, a later blood pressure of 125/85 is much more significant. Practitioners need to monitor pregnant women for toxemia (a serious condition caused by high blood pressure during pregnancy), since it is common during the later months. Toxemia is determined by how much the blood pressure rises, not only by how high it is.

Some women will have preexisting high blood pressure (hypertension) that was undetected before their first prenatal visit. This is because hypertension often has no symptoms and pregnancy is the first time that many women see a doctor regularly. Some doctors will prescribe Aldomet, or a similar medication, to such women to lower their blood pressure. Aldomet has been used for years to treat pregnant women with high blood pressure and has not been shown to harm the development of the fetus.

The practitioner will then check the woman's heart for a loud murmur or irregular heartbeat. Many pregnant women have soft murmurs that are nothing to worry about and are noticed during pregnancy for the first time.

Next, the thyroid gland on the throat is examined to see if it is too large or too small, indicating a problem with thyroid functioning. Many otherwise healthy women have thyroid disease and it is usually not a problem as long as they take care of it.

After examining the upper half of the body, which usually includes a breast exam, the woman lies down on the examining table. She should have an empty bladder so that this exam, and a transvaginal ultrasound, can be done properly. The practitioner feels the abdomen to see if the uterus is the expected size for that many weeks of pregnancy, and a pelvic exam is done using a speculum and gloved fingers. A Pap smear is also done if the woman hasn't had one during the past year. Otherwise, Pap smears are not usually done until at least six weeks after delivery. Many doctors do a transvaginal ultrasound now. It confirms how far along the pregnancy is, in case there is a question later as to whether or not a woman is beyond her expected delivery date or might be delivering prematurely. Early ultrasound also gives information about how healthy the baby is.

Blood Tests

After the physical exam is over, the practitioner will draw a few tubes of blood. The blood will be checked to make sure the woman is not anemic. If she is, she will be advised to get adequate iron. If she is anemic and her red blood cells are small, she may have a condition called thalessemia minor. If her partner also has the same condition, they have a 25 percent chance of having a baby with a rare, devastating disease called thalessemia major, or Mediterranean anemia. It is most prevalent among people of Italian or Greek descent.

Platelets are blood cells that make bleeding stop and cause clotting when there is a wound. The woman's platelets are counted so the practitioner can see if the woman has a chronic condition called idiopathic thrombocytopenic purpura (ITP), which can cause problems. This count also gives information about how to interpret platelet counts later in pregnancy. It is not unusual for a platelet count to drop later in pregnancy for reasons that are not of concern, but if it suddenly plummets, it can be a sign of severe toxemia. The woman's blood is also checked for signs of liver and kidney health. These may be poor without the woman having any symptoms. When that happens, both the mother and baby can suffer. When these problems are diagnosed, the doctor may be able to make the pregnancy safer.

The mother's blood type and antibodies are also determined. If she is Rh-negative, meaning she lacks the Rh protein, her partner's blood type will be checked, too. If his is Rh-positive, meaning he has that protein, she will need a Rhogam injection. If she already has Rh antibodies, it is too late for the injection and she will follow the protocol discussed later in this book (see "Rh Disease" on page 154). While some maternal antibodies are lethal to a baby, the availability of Rhogam has made it rare to have problems due to the mother's Rh antibodies.

The woman's immunity to rubella is checked. If she had rubella, she will be immune for life. If she had the vaccine, it might have worn off by the time she got pregnant. If so, she should try to avoid being around children who might carry it. While rubella vaccines are not given during pregnancy, she will be advised to get one shortly after delivery.

Many states requires pregnant women to be tested for hepatitis B as well. If a pregnant woman is known to have it, her baby will get shots soon after delivery that will prevent it from getting hepatitis from the mother.

If the woman's blood test shows that she has syphilis, she will be treated with antibiotics.

The majority of states require testing the mother for HIV. It is well known that giving anti-HIV medication to the mother decreases the baby's chance of getting the disease.

Most practitioners will then tell the woman things to avoid. These include: drinking alcohol; eating unpasteurized dairy products, uncooked soft cheeses, hot dogs, delicatessen-prepared foods with mayonnaise; taking long, hot baths or using a hot tub; going scuba diving, skiing, or Rollerblading; taking Imitrex for migraines, or using medications that can cause birth defects.

They will discuss future tests and visits, which may include the following office appointments:

At 7 weeks—Taking a medical history, getting a sonogram that shows the fetal heartbeat, and blood tests.

At 11 weeks—Listening for a fetal heartbeat.

At 15 weeks—Doing an alpha-fetoprotein 4 blood test in the office or an amniocentesis in the hospital.

At 19 weeks—Getting a detailed sonogram.

At 24 weeks—Having a glucose challenge test.

At 28 weeks—Women with Rh incompatibility will get Rhogam.

At 32 and 34 weeks—Office visits.

At 36 weeks—A group B strep culture is done. Visits are weekly thereafter until delivery.

The practitioner may also describe what to expect throughout the pregnancy and prescribe prenatal vitamins. He or she might also give literature or a book that includes the above information.

You might ask if your practitioner has a recommended schedule of visits and tests, and what you should do if you experience bleeding, your water breaks, or you have contractions. This is the time to ask other questions that you might have about your practitioner, and to find out with which hospital or birthing center he or she is affiliated.

Find out your practitioner's normal office hours and times that he or she returns patients' routine telephone calls. Unless you have an emergency, these are the best times to contact your practitioner if you have questions or problems between visits.

High-Risk Pregnancy

Because most women have uneventful pregnancies and deliver healthy babies, when are doctors concerned that a woman is "high risk," and what does that mean?

A woman who has a higher than normal chance of having medical complications during pregnancy, and/or of having a baby with problems, may be considered high risk. The Society of Maternal-Fetal Medicine recommends that women consider consulting a high-risk pregnancy specialist when they have any of the following conditions: kidney disease, a multifetal pregnancy, chronic high blood pressure, diabetes, HIV, asthma, lupus, hepatitis, thyroid disease, cardiac disease, genetic disorders, or a history of preterm labor or premature rupture of membranes. A maternal-fetal specialist may also be consulted for prenatal diagnosis with ultrasound and chorionic villi sampling (CVS). Most competent obstetricians can handle the majority of the above-mentioned conditions in conjunction with a qualified internist, endocrinologist, or maternal-fetal specialist.

Other factors that contribute to a riskier pregnancy include smoking cigarettes or drinking alcohol during pregnancy, as well as conditions such as epilepsy, preexisting medical conditions, having been toxemic in a prior pregnancy, or having had a baby who died at birth or who had brain damage. Women who are older than thirty-nine or younger than sixteen are also considered to have higher than normal risk.

Some medical authorities recommend making an initial assessment of a pregnant woman's risk during her first prenatal visit, and repeat it at twenty-eight to thirty weeks of pregnancy. This reassessment is done because some women who are initially low risk become higher risk as the pregnancy continues.

Pregnant women who are high risk should plan to deliver in a hospital with a well-staffed maternity unit, with operating rooms and blood products that are readily available should the need arise. The hospital nursery should also be set up to care for sick or premature babies.

Having Babies after Age Thirty-five

More and more women in the Western world are having their first babies in their thirties or forties, often because they first want to finish their education and get vocationally and financially established. It was estimated that in the year 2000, one out of every twelve American babies was born to a mother who is thirty-five or older.

While some research argues that older mothers don't have any specific risk factors once they do get pregnant, we disagree. We consider mothers thirty-five and older to have higher risks than younger mothers, although with good care all mothers can have an excellent chance of having good pregnancies and healthy babies.

Specifically, mothers over thirty-five are more likely than younger mothers to have high blood pressure and other medical problems when they get pregnant. Mothers over thirty-five also have a greater risk of miscarrying before the twentieth week of pregnancy than younger women do. In fact, women forty-two and older have up to a 70 percent chance of miscarrying.

Chromosomal anomalies such as Down syndrome is the only birth defect believed to increase with the mother's age. A twenty-year-old woman has a 1.9 in 1,000 chance of giving birth to a baby with a chromosomal problem such as Down syndrome. A thirty-year-old woman has a 2.6 in 1,000 risk. A thirty-six-year-old woman has a 5.2 in 1,000 risk. A forty-year-old woman has a 15.2 in 1,000 risk, and a forty-five-year-old has a 47.6 in 1,000 risk. While older mothers certainly have a greater individual chance of having babies with abnormal chromosomes, the statistics can also be viewed another way. While a twenty-year-old woman has more than a 99 percent chance of having a baby with normal chromosomes, a forty-five-year-old has more than a 95 percent chance of having a healthy baby.

In view of the above, we recommend that older women be well prepared and discuss with their practitioner any areas of concern before they get pregnant. The woman should be checked to make sure that her blood pressure, blood sugar, and weight are normal before getting pregnant. High blood pressure, diabetes, or other medical conditions should be well controlled before getting pregnant. If a woman gets pregnant having preexisting medical conditions, most (except for diabetes) will not compromise the early embryo.

In addition, older women should ideally start taking prenatal vitamins that include .8 mg of folic acid before they get pregnant. Women who have not done that should not worry because most will have enough folic acid to prevent birth defects.

While much research has been done on older women who have had babies, little is known about the relationship between the age of the father and its effects on the baby. It is believed that fathers being forty-five or older does not raise the risk of the woman having medical or surgical complications in pregnancy; nor does it increase the chances of having a baby with most chromosomal abnormalities.

A couple with concerns about having a baby with genetic problems should get genetic counseling prior to getting pregnant. A counselor or a specialist in high-risk pregnancy can discuss each couple's risks for having a baby with specific types of birth defects. The specialist can also recommend tests prior to conception, or during pregnancy, to determine if the baby has, or is likely to have, a particular disorder.

Fathers during Pregnancy

Men have an incredible variety of responses to pregnancy and childbirth, just as women do. Some are fascinated by the whole process, from the time they first see their baby's tiny heart beating on a sonogram to the time their newborn emerges into the world. They accompany their wives on every prenatal visit and want to be a part of everything that happens. They coach and support their wives during labor and delivery and take care of the newborn at night.

Some men are repulsed by their wife's expanding girth. Others are more worried about the prospects of having a new set of financial responsibilities than they are about the details of the fetus's development. Still others are happy about the pregnancy, but they don't want to be present during labor and birth because it seems so overwhelming and scary.

Fathers should never be pressured into being present at their baby's birth if they don't want to do so. It may be very upsetting for them to watch their loved one screaming in pain or to see her with tubes and wires connecting her to machines. Since it is important for a laboring woman not to be alone, she should bring a labor coach such as a close friend, mother, or sister for support if possible. A doula (professional labor coach) may also be hired.

Women need to realize that their response to pregnancy may be very different from their husbands'. Women should not assume that a man's lack of enthusiasm during pregnancy will translate into his being a poor father. Many men are much more able to relate to things they can see and touch and talk to than to abstract ideas. Once the strangeness of pregnancy and labor are over, and they hold a baby who looks familiar and precious, these men will probably bond beautifully with their new child and make great fathers.

Sex during Pregnancy

One of the first questions that newly pregnant women grapple with is whether, and how, they must modify their physical intimacy with their partner. It may be difficult for them to broach this with their obstetrical caretakers, but it's important that they do. In a normal pregnancy, it is fine to have sexual intercourse until labor begins or the bag of water breaks. Sex does not hurt the baby, break the bag of water, or cause premature labor. Nor does it cause infections in healthy mothers who have sex with only one man, because the mucus plug in the cervix, together with the cervix and amniotic membranes, prevent the fluids and bacteria in semen from entering the uterus.

Women at high risk for preterm labor, or those who are on bed rest for other reasons, however, should not have sex. This is because semen contains prostaglandins, which can cause the cervix to ripen and bring on uterine contractions. The amount of prostaglandins in male ejaculate is far less than what is needed to endanger a normal pregnancy; this same amount, though, could cause problems for a woman who is at risk for preterm labor.

The same holds true for a pregnant woman having an orgasm or nipple stimulation. Either of these can initiate uterine contractions, and nipple stimulation can even release enough oxytocin to induce labor.

These, and sex, are fine for healthy women with healthy pregnancies, but off-limits for women who have a greater than normal chance of having preterm labor. These are also not okay when a fetus is at risk because the fetus is not growing well.

How do we know that sex is okay for healthy women with healthy pregnancies? A unique study was done at the author's institution in which healthy pregnant women wore monitors while they had sex at home. The monitors showed that stimulating nipples and having an orgasm provoked mild uterine contractions and caused temporary fetal heartbeat irregularities. Some women also said that their babies moved more during intercourse. However, all of these women delivered healthy babies. It was concluded that sex during low-risk pregnancies is fine.

Even though about one-quarter of pregnant women who have orgasms have contractions afterward, these do not usually cause a woman to go into labor. Mild cramping after orgasm usually stops within an hour. If the cramping is more intense than what happens during a menstrual period, or if the cramping doesn't stop within an hour of resting, call your caretaker.

Which pregnant women, then, should abstain? Women who are at high risk for preterm labor because they already had a premature baby after preterm labor, or who were already treated for preterm labor; those with a prematurely dilated cervix; those whose membranes have ruptured; whose placentas have implanted over the cervix (placenta previa); who have blood clots in the uterus; who have had recent vaginal bleeding; or whose fetus could be harmed by even a short period of decreased blood flow to the placenta. Women who are put on bed rest should candidly discuss with their caretakers what specific sexual activities are okay and which must be avoided.

Women for whom having intercourse is okay should still adhere to a few precautions. During the second half of pregnancy (after twenty weeks) women should not lie flat on their backs because the big uterus compresses large blood vessels that deliver blood to the placenta. Instead, they should find positions for intercourse which allow them to be comfortable. Some women find that their added weight makes sex in the missionary position uncomfortable even before twenty weeks. They can try sitting on top of the man while he lays down or sits under her on a bed or sturdy chair. They can lie side by side either facing each other or with the man entering from behind.

Cunnilingus (putting the man's mouth on the woman's genitals) may be done as long as the man does not blow air into the woman's vagina. Blowing air into the vagina can cause air blockages in the woman's bloodstream and lungs, creating a dangerous situation for the mother and baby.

Sexual Feelings during Pregnancy

Many people wonder how other couples feel about having sex during pregnancy, but are too embarrassed to ask. As with other matters, men and women respond to sex during pregnancy in a variety of ways. During the first trimester, a woman's fatigue and nausea, breast soreness, and fears of miscarriage may affect her interest in sex. As pregnancy progresses, many women find that the increased blood flow to their genitals and breasts, along with extra vaginal lubrication, increase their sex drive and responsiveness. Other women feel that their bulky bodies, stretch marks, and bulging veins make them look anything but sexy. Some women also find that the congestion and swelling of their vaginas makes penetration uncomfortable. Back pain and general discomfort during the third trimester may further diminish their sexual interest. Overall, couples have less sex during pregnancy than they did before.

Some couples find that pregnancy makes them feel much closer to each other. The intimacy of having created a baby together heightens their lovemaking. The fact that they don't have to worry about contraception is an added plus.

Some men find a pregnant wife, especially her increased breast size and Rubenesque look, very sexy. On the other hand, men may feel that it's not right to have sex with the mother of their child. They may feel that their penis shouldn't be intruding into the baby's space, or that their wife is now too pure and maternal to be having sex. Others worry that sex will harm the baby or bring on labor.

Unfortunately, some men are simply turned off by the look of a pregnant wife, and this attitude is unlikely to change. A woman, however, should not feel less wonderful about herself because her partner has this negative attitude.

There is not one "right" way to have sex during pregnancy, and couples have a wide range of sexual interest and activity during this time. Some women are content with physical closeness and assurances of their partner's love. As long as it is fine with both partners, complete abstinence is as normal as frequent lovemaking. Pregnant women should not think that they need to be more or less active in order to be "normal."

CHAPTER THREE

Ultrasound

Ultrasound is the use of sound waves to create a picture. These sound waves move much too quickly for the human ear to hear, but they can be harnessed by ultrasound machines into breathtakingly clear pictures. Obstetrical sonograms look like black-and-white photographs taken inside the uterus.

Ultrasound (also called sonogram) is used more in gynecology and obstetrics than in any other branch of medicine, and it has changed obstetrics more than anything else in the history of childbirth. It was widely used in the 1970s, but its technology became much more refined during the 1980s and 1990s. Today, more than 50 percent of American women get sonograms when they are pregnant, and in some places that figure is close to 99 percent!

Until the advent of ultrasound, doctors had to have blind faith that the baby was developing normally. There was no way of being sure of a baby's age, how many fetuses there were, whether or not the placenta was positioned correctly, or whether the baby might have a condition that would require a cesarean section.

Ultrasound allows expectant couples and their caretaker to see the baby, his organs, and his movements as they occur. Because the sound waves used are those above the range that humans can hear, it is considered safe for fetal ears. Studies have not demonstrated any harmful effects of ultrasounds done on the millions of babies who have had them. On the other hand, ultrasound has helped save the lives of countless babies and mothers by revealing problems for which life-saving measures were then used.

An additional benefit of ultrasound is that it helps mothers and fathers bond with their babies even before birth. Parents often place sonogram photos in albums as mementos alongside other precious pictures. It must be mentioned that ultrasound is an expensive medical procedure not to be used unnecessarily. Parents should not get an ultrasound because they want to know the baby's sex so that they can order the right colors for the layette.

How Ultrasound Is Done

There are three possible ways of doing an ultrasound. One is done during the first part (trimester) of pregnancy. Called a transvaginal ultrasound, it involves placing a long probe into the woman's vagina. It sends sound waves through the thin vaginal wall into the uterus. These waves are interpreted into a clear image of the reproductive organs and the developing fetus.

The woman's bladder must be empty when this is done because a full bladder will push aside the organs that are being looked at.

The most common way of doing a sonogram is by putting a transducer against a gel on the expectant mother's abdomen. The instrument sends out sound waves that bounce off different parts of the baby. The reflected waves are then interpreted into images. Bones appear white on an ultrasound screen while amniotic fluid or the baby's urine in its bladder appear black. Tissues like the liver or skin appear as various shades of gray.

This procedure, called a transabdominal sonogram, must be done with a full bladder, making it uncomfortable although not painful.

A translabial ultrasound places a probe against the vulva and vagina in order to give information about the length of the cervix. This is only used in very specific cases where an incompetent cervix or risk of preterm labor are suspected.

Uses of Ultrasound

What are some reasons to use obstetrical ultrasound?

1. *To know how old the baby is*. Ultrasound is the most accurate way of establishing a due date and determining how old the fetus is.

When the fetus is seven to twelve weeks old, ultrasound measures the distance from the top of the head to the bottom of the baby's rump. This measurement can accurately judge the fetal age to within a few days. This is especially useful when a woman has irregular periods, making it difficult to gauge an accurate due date, or when a woman's uterine size is very discrepant from the size it should be according to when she thinks she had her last period. The ultrasound date casts the deciding vote in these cases.

Dating a fetus thirteen to twenty-six weeks old is done by combining the measurements of the distance between the side (parietal) bones of the baby's skull, the distances around the baby's head and abdomen, and the length of its thigh bone (femur). A computer in the ultrasound equipment uses these numbers to estimate the fetal weight with a 10–15 percent margin of error.

The further along the pregnancy is, the less accurately ultrasound predicts the baby's age and weight. Ultrasounds done during weeks thirteen to twenty-six are only accurate to within eight to ten days for estimating fetal age. This is why the due date is not changed when a woman's eighteen- to twenty-week ultrasound gives a due date that is less than ten days discrepant with the date the woman gave. By the end of a pregnancy, the estimated weight might even be off by as much as two pounds.

2. *To know if there is an ectopic pregnancy*. An ectopic pregnancy is one in which the fertilized egg implants and grows outside, instead of inside, the uterus. Typically, the fertilized egg attaches to the thin-walled, more rigid fallopian tube. When the pregnancy reaches a certain size, it will break open the tube and cause internal bleeding. Years ago, women

sometimes died when an ectopic pregnancy ruptured the tube. Today, thanks to ultrasound, a bleeding woman with sharp abdominal pain in one side can be quickly diagnosed and attended to surgically.

3. *To know if the baby will have birth defects known as congenital anomalies.* Ultrasound can see if the ears, arms, forearms, lower legs, and the like are developing normally, and if there are birth defects such as spina bifida or an abnormal heart. Some couples who discover there are anomalies then terminate the pregnancy, while others use the information to prepare for problems that will arise.

Today, some of these defects can be repaired in utero, as when a kidney is blocked and a shunt needs to be placed. Others, such as major heart defects, omphaceles (where part of the intestines stay in the umbilical cord), and abdominal tumors, can be surgically repaired shortly after birth.

Thankfully, today's sophisticated technology allows many babies who would formerly have been severely disabled or dead to do very well. A shunt placed while the baby is in utero can even prevent the kidney from deteriorating.

Ultrasound can also determine when some of the baby's parts are too big or too delicate (such as when there is a large spinal defect) to be safely delivered vaginally.

4. *To see if the baby is alive.* Ultrasound can show if the baby is alive when there is reason to believe that a miscarriage might have occurred. As many as one in three pregnancies ends in a first-trimester miscarriage. Most of these can be detected by the telltale lack of a fetal heartbeat on ultrasound long before other data will confirm the pregnancy loss.

First-trimester ultrasound may be done with women who are anxious because they had a prior miscarriage, those who have had worrisome bleeding, or those whose symptoms of pregnancy (nausea or breast pain) have stopped.

5. *To determine how many babies there are during a multiple pregnancy, whether they are identical or fraternal, how much each weighs, and whether or*

not the difference between them signals problems. Until a few years ago, half of all twin pregnancies were thought to be singletons until the first, smaller than expected, baby was delivered. The existence of the second baby was often as much of a surprise to the doctor as it was to the parents. Lack of knowledge about twins meant that no one paid attention to possible problems the twins might have had during their gestation, let alone during delivery.

Today, routine ultrasound makes the unexpected delivery of twins almost unheard of, and it allows their development to be tracked to make sure they are growing properly.

It matters if the twins will be identical or fraternal because identical twins have a much higher risk than fraternal twins of having complications, usually because of the shared blood supply.

It is especially important for women who conceived with fertility assistance to know how many fetuses are developing. The more fetuses there are, the greater the chance of there being problems. (This is discussed further in the section on multiple births. See page 104.)

6. *To diagnose why a woman is bleeding and to locate the placenta.* Not only can ultrasound show the difference between a healthy pregnancy, an ectopic one, and an impending miscarriage, it can show us the source of bleeding. This can be reassuring when the reason is benign, and life-saving at other times. For example, if ultrasound shows the placenta implanted over the cervix (placenta previa), a cesarean section can be scheduled to avoid tearing the placenta. On the other hand, if it shows that third-trimester bleeding is not being caused by a placenta previa, the obstetrician knows that the woman can be safely examined vaginally.

7. *It allows certain diagnostic tests and fetal therapeutic procedures to be done.* As will be discussed in the chapter on prenatal screening (page 133), amniocentesis and chorionic villi sampling (CVS) can only be done safely when there is ultrasonic guidance. Medical procedures such as blood transfusions to the fetus, fetal kidney shunts, or fixing a blood-flow problem to a twin would also be impossible without ultrasound.

8. *It tells us how big the fetus is so that the practitioner can be prepared when the baby is born.* Certain delivery techniques are used, or avoided, when the baby will be very large or very small. Also, a very small baby might indicate that the mother needs to stop working, stay in bed, or take other measures to try to help the baby grow.

9. *Prior to delivery it tells us what position a baby is in.* When the baby is breech (head-up, buttocks-down) toward the end of pregnancy, ultrasound can be used to help the caretaker turn the baby into a head-down position. If the baby is lying perpendicular to his mother's spine, the mother can be told to call immediately if her bag of water breaks or if contractions start.

10. *It tells us, when women are past their due dates, that the placenta is still functioning, there is enough amniotic fluid, and the baby is still thriving and growing.*

Ultrasounds are also done every two to three weeks throughout the third trimester in high-risk pregnancies to assess fetal growth and well-being.

Forms of Ultrasound

Real-time ultrasound combines still pictures of the fetus much as a cartoonist combines a series of still sketches to create frolicking creatures. One can watch the baby moving, breathing, stretching his limbs, and even sucking his thumb!

The Doppler technique is a type of ultrasound that determines the speed of blood flow in the umbilical cord and/or fetal blood vessels. If the flow is abnormal, it may indicate a delay in nutrients reaching the unborn baby.

A three-dimensional ultrasound allows one to view all three dimensions of the baby in real time. When done by an experienced specialist, this new modality allows very subtle abnormalities to be detected.

*   *   *

Ultrasound is a versatile diagnostic tool that can help practitioners to confirm that a pregnancy is going as expected, reveal problems that may arise, aid in treating such problems, and confirm that a baby is ready (or not) for delivery. It has become such a basic part of the obstetricians' armamentarium that it is hard to imagine the times when a developing fetus was invisible until birth.

CHAPTER FOUR

Physical Changes in Pregnancy

A *woman's body goes through enormous physical changes when she* becomes pregnant. Once the body starts making huge amounts of progesterone, the hormone nourishes the uterine lining while relaxing the uterine muscle. This ensures that the uterus doesn't contract before the baby is ready to be born. Unfortunately for the woman, progesterone also relaxes other smooth muscles in the body besides the uterus, such as the diaphragm, the stomach, and the intestines. When the growing uterus pushes up against the relaxed diaphragm, women can get shortness of breath (dyspnea of pregnancy). This air hunger can be frightening if a woman doesn't understand why it is happening, but it is really no cause for alarm.

During pregnancy, the sphincter muscle of the esophagus relaxes and the stomach below it gets pushed up and compressed. This causes food mixed with stomach acids to be pushed back out of the stomach into the esophagus, causing heartburn. This can be remedied by eating small meals frequently, not eating fatty or spicy foods, and not eating within two to three hours of bedtime. Lying down soon after eating makes the problem worse. Antacids may be taken if they are needed. Those with calcium and without aluminum are best.

Nausea

Most women feel nauseous when they are pregnant, ranging from a queasy feeling that waxes and wanes throughout the day to heaving and vomiting morning until night. It commonly starts at around seven weeks and lasts for another six weeks, although for some women it continues into the second trimester, and a very few vomit daily until they deliver. The term "morning sickness" is really not accurate, because most pregnancy nausea doesn't occur only in the morning. It may be worse when a woman has an empty stomach or a very full one, has eaten oily or spicy foods, or is tired.

What to do about it depends upon how severe it is. If the woman is not losing lots of weight she can be reassured that the problem will stop on its own and will not harm the baby. The baby will get the nourishment it needs from the mother's blood, even if the mother isn't nourishing herself because she feels unwell. Some women find that their prenatal vitamins make them feel worse. They can try taking them in the evening, although they may need to temporarily discontinue them. When that happens, taking .4 mg of folic acid every day is the recommended replacement. Elastic bands, typically used for seasickness, that put pressure on the inside of the wrist help some women, as does acupuncture. Fatigue often aggravates the condition so resting is an obvious solution. Many women find that eating small amounts of foods like rice cakes or whole-grain crackers helps quell the nausea.

Some unfortunate women have hyperemesis gravidarum, or profound nausea and vomiting that is unique to pregnancy. They become dehydrated, lose fifteen to twenty pounds, feel weak and dizzy, and vomit everything they eat. These women need fluids and antinausea medication, usually given in the hospital intravenously at first. Once these women stop vomiting, they may be sent home with oral medication, with nothing, or with an intravenous line that can be taken care of by a specialized nursing service. Very rarely, a woman will need to be fed by infusing nutrients directly into her bloodstream (hyperalimentation).

Women with hyperemesis gravidarum often have it again in subsequent pregnancies, and in some women it gets worse from one pregnancy to the next.

It is not known why pregnant women get nauseous, but it is known that women with multiple fetuses or who have a molar pregnancy get it more than others. (A molar pregnancy is one where the tissue stops developing normally and acts like a tumor.) Both types of pregnancy produce an abnormally high amount of pregnancy hormone (HCG). Still, no one really knows what causes the nausea or what will make it better for all women who have it.

Women who have nausea and/or vomiting during their first trimester often worry that they are starving their baby. After all, the mother is eating poorly, so how well could her baby be faring?

Fortunately, apart from the mother needing a good supply of folic acid for the first six or seven weeks, the fetus during the first trimester does not depend on the mother's diet to survive. It is quite small during this time and it will get all of the nourishment it needs from the mother, even if that means depleting the mother's reserves of vitamins and minerals. Unless the mother loses a considerable amount of weight, and the nausea and vomiting don't stop reasonably soon, some weight loss and a poor diet should not be worrisome during the first trimester.

Constipation

Besides having morning sickness at the beginning of pregnancy, many women suffer from constipation in the latter part of pregnancy. This is because the intestines become sluggish when they are relaxed by progesterone. Women then have more gas and stomachaches, and digested food spends more time in the large intestine. This means that more water is absorbed from the stool before it leaves the body, making pregnant women prone to constipation. The rectum is also compressed as the uterus gets bigger, and this compounds the problem. It is important for pregnant women to drink at least eight glasses of water a day and to make sure their diet contains enough fiber from whole grains, beans, vegetables, and fruits. Stool softeners such as Colace, Metamucil, or Fibercon may sometimes be needed.

Varicose Veins

The body has three types of blood vessels: arteries, veins, and capillaries. It's the job of the arteries to move oxygenated blood from the heart to the rest of the body. Arterial walls are thick and muscular with little "give" to them. As the heart pumps blood through the arteries, the blood quickly shoots to its destinations. The capillaries deliver oxygen and nutrients to the body cells, then the blood returns to the heart for refueling. After leaving the capillaries, the blood goes into the veins but has little force behind it. It relies on the valves in the veins to prevent it from backflowing, especially when it has to move against gravity to get back to the heart—such as in the legs and anus. If one has faulty valves (genes can be blamed for this), the blood pools and stagnates, causing varicose veins. Varicose veins, then, are veins with defective valves.

Many pregnant women develop varicose veins for the first time. The more children women have, and the closer together the pregnancies, the greater the likelihood of getting noticeable varicose veins. Genetics plays a strong role—if your mother had bad varicose veins, you are unlikely to escape them. They get worse as women age, when they stand on their feet a lot, and, most importantly, as they get further along in pregnancy.

Varicose veins can range from purplish fine lines to blue bulges that look like engorged spider webs. They can cause bleeding if they are cut or are traumatized.

It is helpful to elevate the legs higher than the heart as often as possible. Crossing the legs and wearing knee-highs with tight elastic bands just under the knee should be avoided at all costs.

Wearing support hose usually reduces one's pain and discomfort. The hose are put on before getting out of bed in the morning while the woman lies on her back with raised legs. This prevents the blood from pooling in her veins. Regular support hose are available at most drugstores, although some women need them to be specially made at a surgical supply or orthopedic supply store. Neither type improves the condition, and may not prevent it from getting worse, but it usually reduces the pain.

As the uterus grows, it puts pressure on pelvic veins and on the lower part of the main vein of the body (inferior vena cava). This causes the blood to stagnate in the legs and stay away from the brain, resulting in women coming close to fainting or actually fainting when they stand for too long. Lying on one's side will end the fainting spell immediately because it normalizes the blood flow.

Some women get varicose veins in the vulvar area, causing swelling and aching. The pressure makes some women worry needlessly that they are close to labor or that the varicosities will rupture. They needn't worry, as these situations only result in pain.

Thrombosis occurs when blood sits in the veins and clots. This is similar to blood sitting in a test tube or on top of a cut instead of flowing so quickly that is can't "set." When blood clots in the superficial veins of the legs and there is inflammation (thrombophlebitis), it causes pain, and the area is red, hot, and tender. Blood clots of this type rarely break off and cause emboli (clots that travel and block important blood vessels). Affected women are usually advised to elevate their legs, wear support hose when sitting or standing, and apply heat. If there is pain after childbirth, Motrin may be taken.

Deep vein thrombosis is far more dangerous. When blood in the deep veins clots, the clots can break off and block the lungs. A deep vein thrombosis is difficult to diagnose. Sometimes the calf and thigh may feel terribly painful and be swollen, while at other times symptoms are subtle. Prolonged inactivity, like long trips in a car or airplane without getting up and walking every couple of hours, and prolonged bed rest can predispose women to getting deep vein thrombosis.

Women with varicose veins have some swelling and often pain as well. If one leg is painful and swollen, especially where the main vein is at the back, and it wasn't bruised and no muscle was pulled, it should be brought to the attention of one's caretaker.

When women are no longer pregnant, some choose to have a dermatologist or a vascular or plastic surgeon inject their varicose veins with a caustic substance that destroys the diseased veins. Other veins will take over their circulatory function. New varicose veins will develop each year and will likewise need to be injected if a woman wants to eliminate them.

Skin Changes

One of the annoying cosmetic changes during pregnancy is splotchy, irregular brown spots, caused by increased melanin production, that most women get on their faces and necks. We all have melanin, a pigment that makes skin brownish and gives suntans their lovely color. Pregnant women, though, make so much melanin that they may get a raccoonlike appearance called the mask of pregnancy. It is made much worse by staying in the sun.

This extra pigment is also deposited in a line going up from the navel to the chest and down to the pubic bone, as well as in the nipples and genital area, making them darker than usual. Existing scars may also temporarily darken, but this is no cause for alarm. Almost all of the above changes disappear in the months after delivery.

Pregnant women needn't always see a dermatologist if they get numerous skin tags (small, floppy, extra pieces of skin). These are harmless. They proliferate until the baby is born, then go away on their own. On the other hand, certain moles may predispose a woman to getting malignant melanoma. It is important to show your obstetrical caretaker any moles that grow or change during pregnancy. She will know if you need to consult a dermatologist.

Increased estrogen makes the palms redder during pregnancy. If spider veins appear, they often disappear during the three months postpartum. Swollen legs in late pregnancy may look mottled (cutis marmorata), but this also disappears after the baby is born.

A common complaint of pregnant women is stretch marks. These are angry red-purple marks on the abdomen, breasts, and thighs. They seem to be a genetic phenomenon that can't be prevented and may be related to steroid production. (People who take prednisone develop identical marks.) Excessive weight gain makes them worse. Stretch marks fade into silvery-white streaks after delivery, but never entirely disappear.

When the sebaceous glands go into overdrive during pregnancy, some women experience adolescent-type acne. Not much can be done for it, and it is imperative not to use Accutane because it can cause birth defects. Some women use topical clindamycin or erythromycin instead.

Women also may get strange little bumps around their nipples when the modified sebaceous glands enlarge there. These harmless bumps are called tubercles of Montgomery.

Itching

Many women feel itchy, without an associated rash, especially late in pregnancy. If it is so bad that it interrupts sleep and requires taking a shower in the middle of the night for relief, call the practitioner in the morning. Severe itching is sometimes benign cholestasis of pregnancy, a harmless condition for the mother but one that can be associated with problems for the baby. It is due to a temporary obstruction of bile in the liver, and it goes away after birth. The obstruction causes bilirubin (a component of fluid from the gallbladder) to rise, which in turn causes itching and sometimes jaundice.

If you get severe itching, don't panic. A blood test will show if you have increased bilirubin. If so, the fetus will be monitored carefully.

Women occasionally develop an awful pink rash on the abdomen. It may start around the stretch marks and spread to the thighs, buttocks, and arms. This rash is profoundly itchy. This often happens to women during their first pregnancy, but appears late in pregnancy. Women can use steroid creams or antihistamines like Benadryl at any time during pregnancy to get relief. If it is very severe, oral steroids might be needed. Luckily, the rash usually goes away within a week after delivery and rarely recurs with any intensity.

Hair Changes

Pregnant women often find that their hair becomes thicker during pregnancy because the hair that would normally fall out doesn't. In fact, they often have more hair altogether on their face, abdomen, chest, arms, and legs, in the same pattern that men do. The extra body hair goes away after giving birth. Three to six months later they are shocked to find gobs of hair in their hairbrush and in the shower after shampooing. All that extra hair on the head is now falling out months later than it ordinarily should have.

Breast Changes

Many, though not all women, get enlarged and sore breasts during early pregnancy. Wearing a well-fitting bra can minimize the pain. Although the breasts will get larger with pregnancy, the pain usually goes away after the first three or four months.

Some women notice colostrum, the baby's first food, seeping out of their breasts or as crusty material on them. This is perfectly normal.

Eye Changes

It is unusual for significant changes to occur to the eyes during pregnancy, although the cornea does tend to thicken a little because it swells with water. This can cause minor visual changes and some difficulties wearing contact lenses while pregnant.

Abdominal Changes

As a woman's uterus grows, it leans to one side or the other and pushes everything out of its way. In most women, the uterus leans to the right, so many women feel a pulling sensation in their left groin. This stretches the round ligaments that connect the sides of the uterus to the wall of the abdomen. Sudden movements like sneezes or coughs may cause a brief, sharp pain in the lower abdomen.

As many women know, the bladder has less room to store urine as the growing uterus compresses it. Many jokes have been made about the fact that during the latter part of pregnancy, the woman's first concern is proximity to the bathroom. She makes more frequent and not-so-fruitful trips to the bathroom as she nears delivery.

Pregnant women undergo many changes. Reading books such as this can help you distinguish normal changes from worrisome ones. If you are still concerned that something seems too different, consult your health care provider.

CHAPTER FIVE

Nutrition during Pregnancy

*O*ne of the many miracles of pregnancy is that, with the exception of one cell from the father, an entire baby develops from the mother's body. Since the baby has no other nutritional source, it is critical that the mother eat a healthy diet during pregnancy.

You may not be able to change the genes that you give your baby, but you can give it the best chance to be healthy by choosing carefully what you eat when you are pregnant.

Weight Gain

A common fallacy among many pregnant women today is that the more they eat, the healthier the baby will be. Women expecting a single baby need to gain only about twenty-five pounds during pregnancy, though an underweight woman may gain up to thirty-five pounds. This weight is accounted for as follows: The average baby weighs about seven and a half pounds. The placenta weighs one and a half pounds, the amniotic fluid weighs two pounds, the extra uterine tissue weighs two and a half pounds, the breasts gain another two pounds, and extra blood and body fluid add another six to seven pounds. The remaining pounds are deposited as fat on the buttocks, thighs, and abdomen to make sure there is adequate energy for the baby.

Women should gain only two to three pounds during the entire first trimester (thirteen weeks), with about one pound added each subsequent week until the baby is born. Gaining more weight than that serves no constructive purpose, and it may cause health problems for the mother and make it hard for her to lose the excess fat later.

Counting calories is a good way to make sure women don't overeat. The average pregnant woman needs to eat only 2,100 or so calories a day. This is only about 300 calories a day more than she eats when not pregnant. If she eats more calories than she needs, the excess will be converted into fat.

Unfortunately, at least 30 percent of Americans are now obese. Pregnant women who are obese have a greater-than-normal chance of getting gestational diabetes, chronic high blood pressure, toxemia, and blood clots in the legs. It also makes childbirth more difficult and causes problems during labor. It is therefore very important for women to eat healthily and not overeat during pregnancy.

Food Choices

What kinds of nutrients, then, should a pregnant women eat? The same six categories of nutrients that everyone needs, which are proteins, carbohydrates, fats, vitamins, minerals, and water. The first three substances provide energy, while protein also helps to build and repair body organs. The vitamins, minerals, and water are needed for the body to function properly.

The American College of Obstetrics and Gynecology specifically recommends that pregnant women eat foods from six different groupings every day, in the amounts listed below.

1. Carbohydrate-rich foods, such as whole-grain breads or cereals, rice, and pasta. Examples of a portion from this group would be a half cup of any of the following grains: cooked oatmeal, millet, bulghur wheat, brown rice, kasha, quinoa, Wheatena, and the like. Likewise, a slice of whole-grain bread, an ounce of cold cereal (preferably whole-

grain and unsugared), or two ounces of uncooked pasta are a portion. Women are advised to eat six to eleven portions of these daily, or a little more than half of their daily caloric intake.

2. Vegetables, of which a portion is a cup of raw, dark leafy greens such as mixed baby greens (mesclun); romaine, red, or green leaf lettuce; arugula; dandelion greens; or the like. Alternatively, a portion is a half cup of any baked, steamed, or stir-fried vegetable. Asparagus, beet tops, bok choy, broccoli, Brussels sprouts, cabbage, carrots, rutabaga, string beans, summer squash, Swiss chard, zucchini, spinach, kale, mustard greens, and the like are usually steamed or stir-fried. Acorn, buttercup, butternut, and spaghetti squashes are usually baked. Three to five servings a day are recommended.

3. Fruits, of which examples of a portion include an apple, a pear, a peach, half a grapefruit, three-quarters of a cup of orange juice, or a quarter cup of dried fruit. Two to four servings a day are recommended.

4. Dairy products, of which a cup of low-fat milk, eight ounces of yogurt, two ounces of processed cheese, or one cup of cottage cheese are each a portion. Two or three servings a day are recommended.

5. Protein foods include meat, poultry, fish, eggs, nuts, and beans. One portion would be three ounces of tuna fish, three ounces of meat or poultry, one or two eggs, a half cup of beans, a cup of lentils, or a half cup of nuts. Fatty meats, luncheon meats (cold cuts), hot dogs, and fried foods should be avoided. It is best to trim fat off meat and remove skin from poultry before eating. Chicken and fish should be baked, broiled, or steamed. Four to six servings a day are recommended.

6. Fats, oils, and sweets. These should be eaten sparingly. Fat from meats and dairy should not make up more than 10 percent of the daily caloric intake. The best sources of fats are those that occur naturally in fish and the best oils are those found in seeds, nuts, and nontropical plants. Foods with added sugar, such as candies, jelly, cakes, pies, cookies, soft drinks, and sweetened fruit drinks should be avoided.

Pregnant women also need to drink at least eight glasses of water a day.

What Nutrients Do

Why do we need different categories of nutrients? Every person needs more than sixty vitamins, minerals, and amino acids in order to function properly. Just as a car needs fuel to run, and it can't run well with watered-down or contaminated fuel, our bodies can't either. The better the quality of a diet, the better we fuel our bodies to work well. Similarly, just as a car needs all of its parts to work in balance, so do we need balanced combinations of many nutrients, not simply a few here and there. If a car has a full tank of gas but no oil, no transmission fluid, and no brake fluid, it still won't run properly. When we miss even a few important nutrients, entire chains of events in our bodies can break down.

Our bodies depend upon food to give us energy as well as to provide the materials for essential chemical reactions to take place. We have hundreds of enzymes that help the body run properly. None of these enzymes can work efficiently without minerals. Vitamins and hormones also need minerals to function. If we don't get enough proper minerals in the right balance, our body's systems will function poorly, if at all.

Proteins are broken down by the body into substances called amino acids, which are rearranged into new proteins. These enable a body to grow. While nonpregnant women need only 44 grams of protein a day, so much growth occurs during pregnancy that an expectant mother needs 74 grams of protein daily.

Carbohydrates are needed to supply energy, and they are burned up more quickly than protein or fat. Carbohydrates include sugars and starches, as well as the indigestible fiber that helps prevent constipation. Pregnant women need to eat 25 grams of fiber every day.

A small amount of dietary fat is needed to absorb fat-soluble vitamins, facilitate digestion, and maintain health of the nervous system.

Vitamins

There are two basic kinds of vitamins: some are water-soluble, like the B vitamins and vitamin C, while others are fat-soluble, like vitamins A, D, and E. The water-soluble vitamins are heat sensitive and easily destroyed by cooking. Foods containing them should be cooked only briefly, in a minimum of water.

Fat-soluble vitamins should be taken in a fatty form, such as oil in a capsule, or they should be eaten after foods that contain fat. Because our bodies store these vitamins, it is possible to get toxic amounts of vitamins A or D if huge amounts are taken over a long period of time.

Vitamin A
800 milligrams daily

Vitamin A helps the cells to grow and develop and tissues to heal. It is needed for the bones and teeth to form, and for healthy skin, hair, mucous membranes, and eyes. Good sources are fish liver oils, beef liver, egg yolk, and fortified milk. The body also makes Vitamin A from beta-carotene, a pigment found in orange fruits and vegetables, as well as many green vegetables. Good sources are carrots (especially cooked), sweet potatoes, rutabaga, apricots, cantaloupe, orange squashes, pumpkin, broccoli, and spinach.

B VITAMINS

We need B vitamins to be able to use the calories, or energy, in the food we eat.

Thiamine (B_1)
1.5 milligrams daily

Thiamine, or vitamin B_1, is needed for heart, muscle, and nervous system functioning, as well as for digestion and growth. It keeps the skin, eyes, hair, and mouth healthy. Good sources are organ meats, nuts, wheat germ, poultry, fish, brown rice, legumes, whole grains, blackstrap molasses, beans, sunflower seeds, and collard greens.

Riboflavin (B_2)
1.6 milligrams daily

Riboflavin, or vitamin B_2, is needed for metabolizing food, for making antibodies and red blood cells, and for eye, hair, nail, and skin health. Good sources of vitamin B_2 are liver, milk, yogurt, whole grains, blackstrap molasses, nuts, egg yolks, and cheese.

Niacin (B_3)
17 milligrams daily

Niacin (nicotinic acid), or vitamin B_3, is needed for proper growth, the skin, and nervous and digestive systems. Good sources are beans, green vegetables, dairy, meat, poultry, whole grains, legumes, and nuts.

Pantothenic Acid (B_5)
10 milligrams daily

Pantothentic acid, or vitamin B_5, is needed for making antibodies. It stimulates growth and is good for the skin and adrenal glands. It is found in egg yolks, orange juice, brewer's yeast, legumes, liver, whole grains, mushrooms, salmon, and wheat germ.

Pyridoxine (B_6)
22 milligrams daily

Pyridoxine, or vitamin B_6, is needed to metabolize our food and control weight. It is good for healthy skin, nerves, and muscles; digestion; and making antibodies. Deficiency can cause anemia, irritability, skin disorders, muscle problems, depression, and hair loss. The more protein one eats, the more B_6 one needs. Good sources are milk, cabbage, cantaloupe, blackstrap molasses, whole grains, prunes, leafy green vegetables, meats, fish, poultry, shellfish, and legumes.

Cobalamin (B_{12})
2.2 milligrams daily

Cobalamin, or vitamin B_{12}, is essential for making red blood cells, keeping nerve cells healthy, and metabolizing food. Getting too little vitamin B_{12} can cause a form of anemia, with fatigue, weakness, and poor appetite. Good sources are liver, meat, fish, eggs, dairy products, miso, tempeh, and sea vegetables.

OTHER ESSENTIAL VITAMINS

Biotin (Vitamin H)

No minimum daily requirement during pregnancy has been established

Biotin (vitamin H) promotes growth and helps us store carbohydrates and make fat. It helps make healthy hair, skin, and muscles. It is found in sardines, liver, legumes, egg yolks, brown rice, lentils, mung bean sprouts, whole grains, and organ meats.

Choline

No minimum daily requirement has been established

Choline is needed to keep our nerves healthy and help our bodies use fat and cholesterol. It is good for the hair and thymus gland. It is found in leafy green vegetables, lecithin, egg yolks, fish, legumes, organ meats, soybeans, and wheat germ.

Folic Acid

.4 milligram daily

Folic acid, also called folate, is needed to make new cells and some enzymes, and for cells to grow and reproduce. It is good for the glands and liver. Adequate amounts provide good protection against having babies with neural tube defects. Good sources include root vegetables, tuna, dairy products, organ meats, cooked oysters, salmon, cooked spinach, leafy green vegetables, legumes, whole grains, and orange juice.

Women who took certain medications, including antacids, or who regularly drank alcohol or smoked cigarettes prior to getting pregnant have higher needs for folic acid. Therefore, while most pregnant women need only 400 micrograms a day, it is recommended that women take 800 micrograms (.8 milligram) of folic acid prior to and during at least the first two months of pregnancy.

Inositol

No minimum daily requirement has been established

Inositol is critical for hair growth, metabolizing fats and cholesterol, and making lecithin. It is also good for the development of vital organs. It is found in citrus fruits, nuts, milk, meat, blackstrap molasses, whole grains, vegetables, and lecithin.

Para-aminobenzoic Acid (PABA)
No minimum daily requirement has been established
Para-aminobenzoic acid (PABA) is needed to break down and use protein and to form red blood cells. It promotes growth, helps bacteria make folic acid, and keeps the skin and hair healthy. It is found in leafy green vegetables, organ meats, yogurt, wheat germ, and blackstrap molasses.

Ascorbic Acid (Vitamin C)
No minimum daily requirement has been established
Ascorbic acid, or vitamin C, is needed for the body to make amino acids, collagen, and thyroid hormone. It is an antioxidant and strengthens the immune system and blood vessels. It keeps teeth, bones, and gums healthy and helps the body make collagen. Good sources are citrus fruits, tomatoes, alfalfa sprouts, papaya, cantaloupe, peppers, berries, green leafy vegetables, broccoli, cauliflower, cabbage, and some sea vegetables.

Calciferol (Vitamin D)
5 micrograms daily
Calciferol, or vitamin D, is needed for building bones and teeth and keeping the nervous system healthy. It is good for the thyroid gland and normal blood clotting. It can be gotten from casual exposure to outdoor sun for twenty to thirty minutes several times a week, as well as from fortified milk, egg yolks, herring, sardines, tuna, salmon, and fish liver oil.

Tocopherol (Vitamin E)
10 milligrams daily (if taken in supplements, it should be in the form of d-alpha tocopherol)
Tocopherol, or vitamin E, is needed to break down oxidants that destroy cell membranes. It protects fat-soluble vitamins and red blood cells, prevents blood clots, keeps the muscles and nerves healthy, and strengthens the capillaries. It is also good for the hair, skin, and mucous membranes. Good sources are wheat germ; cold-pressed, unrefined oils; almonds; and hazelnuts.

Unsaturated Fatty Acids (omega-3, omega-6, linolenic acid, vitamin F)

No daily minimum requirements have been established

Unsaturated fatty acids, which include omega-3, omega-6, and linolenic acid (vitamin F), are needed for healthy skin and normal cellular and glandular activity. These fatty acids destroy cholesterol, prevent hardening of the arteries, and regulate blood coagulation. Essential fatty acids are unsaturated fats that we must get in our diet because our bodies cannot manufacture them. While people tend to associate the word *fats* with heart disease, essential fatty acids are necessary for normal brain and eye development in infants and toddlers, and they are necessary throughout life for the normal functioning of the body. The best ratio of omega-3 to omega-6 is about six to one. Good sources of fatty acids are unrefined, cold-pressed oils; flaxseed, borage, and evening primrose oils; wheat germ; nuts and sunflower seeds; and cold-water fish such as salmon and herring.

When fish such as salmon are commercially farmed, they have only about one-third as much omega-3 as those that grow in the wild. This is because farmed fish are fed a diet of grain instead of the plankton and algae that make the omega-3 oils that accumulate in wild fish.

Phylloquinone (Vitamin K)

65 micrograms daily

Phylloquinone, or vitamin K, is needed to form prothrombin for blood coagulation, as well as for healthy liver functioning. Good sources are cauliflower, soybeans, polyunsaturated oils, fish liver oils, egg yolk, yogurt, kelp, leafy green vegetables, blackstrap molasses, and alfalfa.

Bioflavonoids

No daily minimum has been established

Bioflavonoids like rutin and hesperidin (vitamin P) are needed for cold and flu resistance, for protection against bruising, and for healthy capillary walls and connective tissue. They are found in buckwheat (kasha), black currants, cherries, grapes, and other fruits.

Minerals

Following are some of the more commonly known minerals, a summary of what they do, and where they are found:

Calcium
1,000 milligrams daily

Calcium is one of the best-known minerals, since it is the major building block of bones and teeth. It is also needed for muscle and nerve functioning and for blood clotting, normal blood pressure, and prevention of osteoporosis. Milk and dairy products are the best-known sources, although these are not tolerated by some people.

Excellent nondairy sources of calcium include fortified soymilk, canned fish with bones, broccoli, dark leafy greens, sesame and sunflower seeds, tahini, chickpeas, blackstrap molasses, tofu, almonds, figs, sea vegetables, and some herbal teas such as nettles and mint.

Chromium
No minimum daily requirement has been established

Chromium improves the effectiveness of insulin in regulating blood sugar, stimulates enzymes in energy metabolism, and is needed to synthesize fatty acids, cholesterol, and proteins. Good sources are whole grains, clams, brewer's yeast and unrefined corn oil.

Copper
No minimum daily requirement has been established

Copper is part of many enzymes and is needed to form elastin and red blood cells. Too little copper may result in general weakness and skin sores. Good sources of copper are soybeans, raisins, nuts, organ meats, fish, legumes, and blackstrap molasses.

Iodine
175 micrograms daily

Iodine regulates energy production and metabolism rate, helps thyroid function, prevents goiter, and is needed for healthy nails, skin, teeth, and hair. Good sources are ocean fish, sea salt, and sea vegetables.

Iron
30 milligrams daily

Iron is needed to build muscle, for the blood to carry oxygen, and for the body to use energy. Good sources are a grainlike seed called teff, liver, clams, meat, poultry, egg yolk, legumes, blackstrap molasses, fish, leafy dark green vegetables, dried apricots, seaweeds, spinach, potatoes, raisins, prunes, nuts, seeds, and whole grains. Iron is best absorbed when taken with vitamin C. If it is taken in pill form, it should be taken on an empty stomach, and it should not be taken with zinc and calcium.

Magnesium
300 milligrams daily

Magnesium is needed with calcium and phosphorus for bones to mineralize, for teeth to stay healthy, for muscles to contract, and for nerve impulses to be transmitted. Good sources include nuts, legumes, whole grains, dark green vegetables, and seafood.

Phosphorus
700 milligrams daily

Phosphorus is needed with calcium to build bones and teeth. It is also needed in all of the body cells. Together, calcium and phosphorus make up three-quarters of the total weight of minerals in the body. While calcium deficiency is common, phosphorus deficiency is rare.

Potassium
No minimum daily requirement has been established

Potassium affects the heart muscles, nervous system, and kidneys. It is important in maintaining normal blood pressure. Potassium works in balance with sodium. Good sources are meats, whole grains, legumes, dried fruits, dates, figs, bananas, apricots, nuts, and seafood.

Selenium
65 micrograms daily

Selenium works with vitamin E. It preserves tissue elasticity and is needed for protein utilization. Good sources are broccoli, onions, tuna, herring, wheat germ and bran, whole grains, and brewer's yeast.

Zinc
15 milligrams daily

Zinc is needed for normal growth and development of tissues, bones, and the fetal brain. It's also necessary for our senses of smell and taste. It's involved in immune reactions and needed for sperm production. Good sources of zinc are oysters, organ meats, fish, whole grains, beans, soybeans, and sunflower seeds. Taking iron pills can reduce zinc absorption.

There is no one single pill that can provide all of the nutrients that a woman needs every day. The United States Public Health Service recommends that pregnant women take extra folate, vitamins B_6, C, and D, calcium, copper, iron, and zinc because they are typically deficient in these nutrients.

Vegetarian Diets

Some pregnant women prefer to eat no animal products. If they do this, they should make sure to get enough complete protein and vitamin B_{12} in their diets. One can get B_{12} from tempeh, miso, sea vegetables, or a vitamin supplement. Vegetarian foods containing large amounts of protein include soybeans (which are really legumes), beans, peas, nuts, seeds, peanut and almond butters, and quinoa (a grain). For example, plain soymilk contains from 6 to 10 grams of protein, two tofu hot dogs contain 18 grams, a serving of whole-wheat pasta contains 7 grams, two tablespoons of almond butter contain 8 grams, and a mere four ounces of tempeh (a food made from soybeans) contains 20 grams of protein, along with 100 milligrams of calcium and 6 milligrams of iron.

Variety and Minimally Processed Foods

While it is important to eat carbohydrates, it is best to avoid refined foods such as white bleached flour and white rice. Unless the label on flour says unbleached, it is usually bleached with a chemical like Clorox. Bleaching strips away most of the whole wheat's twenty or so nutrients, including removing 75 percent of the magnesium, 93 percent of the fiber, 50 percent of the linolenic acid and essential fatty acids, and all of its vitamin E. Whole wheat, wheat germ, and even unbleached white flour are better choices. White rice has likewise been stripped of most of its nutrients. Brown rice is a much more nutritious choice.

Cooking vegetables at a high heat and processing, packaging, and storing foods for a long time all destroy much of the vitamins. Fresh foods will nourish your body more than canned or packaged foods will; foods that are minimally cooked are more nourishing than those whose nutrients were affected by boiling or overcooking. In addition, a varied, healthful diet is more likely to give you more of the nutrients you need than eating the same few foods day in and day out.

Fats

Avoid purified cooking oils, especially cottonseed, which is sometimes listed on labels simply as "vegetable oil." These oils have been processed with strong chemicals that leave residues and remove most of the nutrients. Since cottonseed oil is not considered a food (although it is commonly used in food products), it may contain levels of pesticides not approved for food.

Commercially prepared fried foods such as doughnuts, egg rolls, French fries, fried chicken, and fried Chinese food in restaurants are cooked in refined oil that is heated to very high temperatures, then may be reused for several days. This often makes the oil rancid and contains substances called free radicals, which can cause cellular damage. These deep-fried foods also contain too much fat.

It was once thought that margarine was far healthier than butter. We now know that eating hydrogenated fats puts women at risk for heart disease and other health problems. Besides margarine, foods containing hydrogenated fats typically include cakes, cookies, pies, biscuits, candy and granola bars, some breads, some mayonnaises, soups, frozen dinners, and sauces and gravies. If a food label says a product contains hydrogenated or partially hydrogenated fat, look for a healthier alternative that uses a small amount of butter or unrefined oil.

Sweets

The average American ingests more than three-fourths of a cup of sugar a day! Limit foods such as sugared cereals, soft drinks, sweetened fruit drinks, pies, cakes, candies, cookies, pancakes or waffles with syrup, ice creams, frozen yogurt, sweetened yogurts, chocolate milk, desserts like rice pudding and custard, candied sweet potatoes, and the like.

Most of these foods can be made healthfully without sugar. For example, rice pudding can be made using brown rice and milk or enriched vanilla soymilk, with raisins added for sweetness. Fresh fruit, stewed or raw, is a healthier alternative to conventionally prepared pies. Plain, fat-free yogurt can be blended with fresh fruit as an alternative to presweetened yogurt, or a smoothie can be made out of fresh fruit and milk or yogurt instead of drinking a sugary milkshake. Small amounts of orange juice or apple juice concentrate also make nice sweeteners.

Beverages

Pregnant women should be sure to drink plenty of water every day. Minimize drinking caffeinated and soft drinks. Also, avoid drinking acidic beverages out of pottery glazed with leaded paints that were made outside the United States.

If your drinking water at home and at work are not safe to drink, buy bottled water that comes from an unpolluted source, or use a water filter. Activated charcoal filters will take out chlorine, pesticides, industrial solvents, and radon gas, but only a reverse osmosis unit will take out nitrates or lead.

Produce

Today, many people prefer to buy organically grown produce because most conventionally grown foods are sprayed with pesticides and other chemicals whose effects on fetal health is not known. Produce such as berries and potatoes are also coated with fungicides. Many other fruits and vegetables are coated with shellac or petroleum-based waxes to keep them from spoiling. In addition, studies have shown that organically grown produce is usually much more nutritious than that which is conventionally grown.

When conventionally grown fruits and vegetables are bought, some experts from the Environmental Protection Agency advocate peeling them, if possible, to remove some of the chemicals. If that isn't practical, scrubbing and rinsing unwaxed produce with water is better than doing nothing. If they are waxed, it is best to peel them.

Much of the produce that the United States imports from countries such as Mexico and South America contains more pesticide residue than that which is domestically grown. These may include vegetables such as tomatoes, asparagus, broccoli, and spinach (especially frozen), and fruits such as grapes and mangoes that are imported during the winter.

Dairy Substitutes

At least 20 percent of Caucasians have lactose intolerance, as do 50–97 percent of African-Americans, Hispanics, and Asians. Many of these same people have difficulty digesting casein (milk protein) as well. Others have allergic reactions or irritable bowel syndrome when they drink milk or eat dairy.

Women who would like to get calcium from nondairy sources have many options. Fortified soymilk can be used in place of milk. It can replace milk or cream in soups, milkshakes, on hot or cold cereal, and it makes a great pudding. There are so many soymilk brands and flavors on the market it is easy to find one to suit your taste. It is better to avoid the ones sweetened with cane juice (sugar) or corn syrup and choose those that use barley malt or rice syrup instead.

Tofu is a high-protein soy food that has about half the calcium per serving that cheese has, but far less fat. It has little taste of its own and absorbs the sauces or flavorings in which it is cooked. Many companies that make tofu also print recipe booklets of how it can be used, such as in nondairy cheesecake, stir-fried with vegetables, baked with seasoning, used on pizza, put into casseroles, used in mock egg salad. . . . Tofu has an almost endless variety of ways it can be prepared.

If you are allergic to both dairy and soy, don't panic. Consider a cup of chickpeas, almonds, or canned salmon, or a can of sardines with bones.

Each has more calcium than a cup of milk. Ground-up sesame seeds, tahini, broccoli, kale, and steamed greens are all good sources of calcium, as are sea vegetables.

Sea Vegetables and Sea Salt

Sea vegetables are so incredibly rich in calcium, iron, iodine, and other minerals that one serving a day supplies much of one's mineral needs.

Hiziki, a seaweed that is usually steamed with sautéed onion and carrot and seasoned with sesame oil or soy sauce, has more calcium than any other food and has the added benefit of having more iron than meat. Agar flakes, another form of seaweed, can be used to make Jell-O–type desserts. Wakame is mostly used in soups or salads. Nori can be used to make nori rolls with rice and vegetables. Kombu, a form of kelp, is typically cooked in soups or with beans. It makes beans less gassy and reduces their cooking time.

A cup of most of the cooked seaweeds supplies about 600 milligrams of calcium—about twice that of a glass of milk. They also contain lots of trace minerals, as well as iron and iodine.

Some sea salt contains about 80 percent sodium and about 20 percent trace minerals, including iodine. Regular iodized salt provides only salt and iodine. Using mineral-rich sea salt instead of table salt in cooking and baking can help provide trace minerals.

Food Cravings

It is perfectly normal to have food cravings during pregnancy. The most common one, surprisingly, is the desire for orange juice. Sometimes a craving for one food can be remedied by eating a food that is totally unrelated. For example, some women crave sweets, but they find that eating a high-protein food will take away the urge. At other times, eating sweet vegetables such as butternut squash, rutabaga, sweet potato, or carrots might do the trick. If you have cravings for "junk foods," try experimenting with healthier alternatives and see if they feel satisfying.

CHAPTER SIX

Herbs during Pregnancy

In times past, people used herbs and relied on eating a good diet to keep themselves healthy. Today, 30 percent of all modern conventional drugs are derived from plants, and herbs are used widely. It has been estimated that at least 60 million adult Americans, or more than one in three adults, use herbs for medicinal purposes. They spend more than $5 billion a year on the more than twenty thousand herbs and herbal preparations that are available in the United States.

The field of medicine uses three levels of scientific evidence to substantiate recommendations about how to treat certain problems. Level A recommendations are based on strong scientific evidence, usually based on well-designed studies using many participants. One such example is the finding that treating or preventing high blood pressure can reduce the number of strokes that people have. Level B recommendations are based on limited scientific evidence. Most of the recommendations made in this and other medical books are in this category. Level C recommendations are mostly based on consensus and expert opinions. Even though most recommendations made by alternative medicine, acupuncture, herbal therapy, and the like belong to this category, and some doctors do not endorse herbal therapy, no reference book on pregnancy would be complete without discussing herbs that are widely used.

At the present time, there is a great deal of anecdotal information about how best to use herbs, sometimes based on how they have been used for thousands of years. Recently, the National Institutes of Health has allocated funds to scientifically research some recommendations made by alternative healing groups. Over the next decade we hope to see a number of well-designed studies that can move some Level C recommendations to Levels B and A.

We know that herbs have been used in an attempt to maintain good health and to treat disorders for thousands of years. Some of them have been tested in clinical trials during the past two decades and have been found to be effective. Herbs such as echinacea, St.-John's-wort, palmetto, and hawthorn are currently used by many Americans to try to bolster the immune system, fight depression, maintain prostate health, and lower high blood pressure, respectively. Many herbs are alleged to help women get pregnant and stay healthy during their pregnancies.

Unfortunately, today's American health care provider and consumer are not necessarily informed about potential side effects that herbs can have, when they should not be used, and how they interact with other herbs and medications. Doctors and laypeople in European countries tend to be more knowledgeable about, and reliant on, herbs than they are in the United States. We recommend that any pregnant woman who is contemplating using herbs do so only under the supervision of a skilled caretaker who was trained in use of herbs during pregnancy. We do not recommend that laypeople prescribe herbs for themselves. We have deliberately not included dosages of herbs that are used during pregnancy so that readers will not be tempted to take herbs without appropriate consultation.

Many people have the erroneous impression that herbs are harmless. Nothing could be further from the truth. While many herbs are effective for specific conditions and have no known side effects, other herbs can potentially harm the person taking them or have a detrimental effect on a pregnancy.

Herbs are taken during pregnancy for four purposes:

- To strengthen and nourish the body

- To help the body deal with other, unrelated problems, such as allergies and colds

- To prevent miscarriage or preterm labor

- To prepare the body for labor and delivery

Herbs are sometimes taken inadvertently by pregnant women who drink herbal teas and dietary supplements. It is important to be aware of how these herbs can affect pregnancy.

Misconceptions about Herbs

First, many people expect herbs to be miracle drugs that will make them feel better immediately. In fact, many herbs have a very gradual effect on the body, and must be used at least once or twice a day for weeks or months before their effect is noticeable. Most herbal programs are designed to treat a whole person's system, not give a quick fix.

Second, herbs can be one aspect of a program for good health during pregnancy. However, taking herbs is not a replacement for eating a good diet, getting enough rest, and taking other necessary precautions during pregnancy.

Third, one doesn't simply "take herbs." There are many different ways to take herbs, and not all are equally effective with every herb. For example, some herbs are best taken in capsules, while taking other herbs this way gives too little of the active ingredients to be useful. Some herbs are taken in alcohol extracts called tinctures, while others are taken as teas. Herbal infusions are made by taking dried plant leaves, steeping them in very hot water, and using the resulting strained tea. Decoctions are made by boiling herb roots and barks.

Fourth, not all herbs of the same variety are equally effective. They must be fresh and of good quality in order to be most effective. How an herb was grown, harvested, and prepared, and how long it has been sitting on a store shelf, has a great deal to do with how potent it will be.

Finally, different practitioners use different herbs to accomplish similar purposes, depending upon which system they use. More than one herb may be effective for the same problem. Some may be more easily found in one area than another, some may be cheaper than others, and some may be more easily tolerated by one individual than by another.

Don't hesitate to ask for alternatives if the herbs recommended are hard to find, expensive, distasteful, or the like.

Herbs That Pregnant Women Should Avoid

When herbs may be harmful to a fetus, the effects are usually most pronounced during the first trimester (thirteen weeks of pregnancy). A cautious approach would recommend that pregnant women not use herbs during the first trimester unless they are needed for a medical condition where herbs are a treatment of choice and they have been prescribed by a skilled herbologist. When extracts of herbs are needed, it is generally preferable for pregnant women to use whole plant extracts instead of concentrated extracts.

Some commonly used herbs may be dangerous to ingest during pregnancy because they may cause fetal problems or spontaneous abortion. Among herbs to be avoided are the following: aloe vera (aloe gel or juice is okay), angelica, anise, arnica, Asian ginseng, black or blue cohosh, blessed thistle, castor, comfrey, dong quai, ephedra, fenugreek, feverfew, large amounts of ginger, gingko, goldenseal, horehound, Job's tears (mugwort), lemongrass, licorice, lobelia, ma huang, poke, red clover, sassafras, saw palmetto, shepherd's purse, Siberian ginseng (avoid especially during first trimester), willow bark, and yellow dock.

Some of these herbs are used to prepare women for labor or delivery, but they should not be used at any other time because they could cause preterm labor or spontaneous abortion. Also, the amounts of licorice that one might eat in candy are not considered dangerous, nor are the amounts of mugwort that one might eat in macrobiotic foods such as mochi.

Although they are all called ginseng, American, Asian, and Siberian ginseng are not the same. They have different properties and the Siberian variety is specifically contraindicated for use during pregnancy. While normal doses of whole ginger are not generally regarded as problematic, concentrated purified ginger is not recommended.

St.-John's-wort is used by many people to treat their depression. Some herbalists think that it should not be used during the first trimester, and are concerned that it might promote preterm labor later in pregnancy.

Dandelion tea should be avoided during the first trimester, but it is a good source of calcium and iron after that.

Tonics

While some herbs may be harmful to a fetus or contraindicated during pregnancy, others have been safely used by women for thousands of years. Some of these herbs help nourish the body, others promote fertility, others are used to prepare the uterus and cervix for labor and delivery, still others are used to stop preterm labor and threatened spontaneous abortion.

Tonics are gentle, nourishing herbs that herbalists consider to be safe. Some women take one to three cups of tonic infusions every day while they are pregnant. Although some of these herbs are available as teas, tinctures (alcohol extracts), and in capsules, most herbalists recommend that they be taken as infusions. Infusions are strong teas made by steeping an ounce or so of herb, or mixture of herbs, in a quart of just-boiled water, then covering the mixture until the tea cools. It is then strained and is either drunk then or refrigerated for later use. Typically, a cup or more of the liquid is drunk every morning and another cup in the evening. Infusions are best used within twenty-four to forty-eight hours of preparation because the active ingredients oxidize over time.

Tonics are often recommended for pregnant women by herbalists and midwives. Apart from the specific effects of some herbs (like red raspberry) on the uterus, tonics supply nutrients such as calcium, magnesium, and iron in a form that is well absorbed. Many women find it easier to drink a cup or two of herbal tea every day than to eat a lot of food that delivers the same amount of nutrients. This may be especially useful for women who have morning sickness and who can drink but not eat.

A cup of the following infusions gives approximately the following amounts of minerals (in milligrams):

	CALCIUM	MAGNESIUM	POTASSIUM
Alfalfa	75	19	100
Dandelion (and 13 mg of iron and 1 mg of zinc!)	240	37	870
Horsetail	57	36	130
Mint	445	192	3,550
Nettles (and 2.5 mg of iron)	229	50	
Oatstraw	119	100	100
Raspberry	101	26	111

Tea made from one teaspoon of dried mint in one cup of water can contain 445 milligrams of calcium, 192 milligrams of magnesium, and 3,550 milligrams of potassium. By comparison, an eight-ounce glass of cow's milk has 250–300 milligrams of calcium, 125–150 milligrams of magnesium, and almost no iron. Cow's milk is also not well tolerated by some.

In addition to providing a significant amount of calcium, red raspberry tea also has a great deal of manganese in it, which has been used to promote fertility. Some herbalists and midwives recommend taking one or two cups daily of red raspberry tea throughout a pregnancy, and as much as three cups a day in the ninth month. Taking more than one cup a day may not be recommended for women who have uterine irritability or who are at risk for preterm labor. Red raspberry has been shown to increase blood flow to the uterus, and can make labor shorter and more efficient.

Nettles provide iron, calcium, vitamin C, and chlorophyll. They seem to help the kidneys filter waste from the blood more effectively and act as a mild diuretic. They may also help reduce edema. In addition, they have been used for their anti-inflammatory properties when a woman has a urinary tract infection.

Dandelion is high in vitamins A, B complex, and C, calcium, iron, potassium, boron, and silicon. It is thought to help digestion and eliminate waste products from the body. Both dandelion and nettles are considered useful in preventing and treating anemia. Dandelion should not be used during the first trimester.

Oatstraw and alfalfa are used to provide nutrients, and spearmint is especially high in calcium.

When herbs are used as tonics during pregnancy, individual ones are usually alternated every few days, or mixtures of herbs are used. For example, a woman might take one or two cups of raspberry tea daily for three or four days, followed by the same amount of oatstraw for four days, followed by the same amount of nettles for four days, then start the cycle again.

Combinations of herbs may also be used where two parts each of nettles, raspberry, and oatstraw are combined with one part of dandelion leaf, spearmint, alfalfa, and other herbs. An infusion is made from an ounce of the combination steeped in a quart of water, and a cup is drunk twice a day. Since some of these herbs taste strong and/or bitter, most women like to sweeten the tea with a bit of stevia (a plant extract that is two hundred times sweeter than sugar), or with a small amount of fruit juice. If a woman is diabetic, her use of juice must be tailored accordingly.

Herbs Used to Prevent Miscarriage

Herbs have been used in attempts to stop preterm labor and uterine contractions that might otherwise result in spontaneous abortions of normal fetuses. Black haw and cramp bark have been shown to stop uterine contractions in some women, and they have been used for centuries by Native Americans to prevent miscarriage and stop preterm labor. These herbs are usually taken as decoctions (infusion-type tea made from the bark instead of the leaves), although tinctures may also be used. It is believed that these herbs will not stop a "defective" pregnancy from terminating when there is a threatened miscarriage, but may stop a healthy fetus from being spontaneously aborted.

These herbs are sometimes taken with a tincture of helonias, also known as false unicorn.

Wild yam is also used in conjunction with other herbs to prevent miscarriage, especially when uterine cramping is a major symptom.

Partridgeberry is also used by some herbalists at any time during pregnancy to stop bleeding, prevent a miscarriage, or stop preterm labor.

A tincture of the berries of vitex agnus castus, also known as chasteberry, is sometimes used to maintain adequate progesterone levels during the first trimester in women who have had first-trimester miscarriages. A commercially available extract of chasteberries is called Agnolyt.

When women have had prior miscarriages, a tincture of black haw, partridgeberry, and wild yam may be recommended starting two to three weeks before the gestational age at which the prior miscarriages happened, and continuing for a few weeks afterward.

Herbs Used to Prepare for Labor and Delivery

Herbs that are used to prepare the woman's body for labor and delivery are usually taken no earlier than thirty-six weeks' gestation. Some herbalists recommend taking tinctures of the following three herbs daily during the last month of pregnancy:

Black cohosh tincture is used, alone or in combination with other herbs, to prepare for labor or to initiate labor contractions. Black and blue cohosh have been shown to cause uterine contractions, but if the quality and dose are not carefully monitored, too much may be taken and complications may result. Cottonroot bark tincture may be used during labor to increase the effect of oxytocin that is already in the woman's body. A decoction of partridgeberry may be taken during the last month of pregnancy to make labor easier and faster.

Evening primrose oil is currently being used by some women who are overdue who hope to avoid the need for induced labor. It contains linoleic acid, which is a precursor of misoprostol, a chemical that causes cervical ripening, which, hopefully, then leads to labor. Evening primrose oil is currently being investigated to see if its use results in higher rates of cesarean sections.

Herbs Used for Medical Problems during Pregnancy

Tinctures of red root and ginger are sometimes taken along with echinacea tincture to ward off a cold or flu or to reduce its severity. Red root and echinacea are used to reduce symptoms of a sore throat when the lymph nodes are swollen.

A great deal of research, both clinical and anecdotal, has shown that elderberry flower tea or a syrup made from elderberries can strengthen the immune system and increases resistance to influenza and other viruses. It has been shown to reduce the time of recuperation from viruses, especially the flu, as well as to reduce the incidence of viral infections among people who took it as compared with placebo.

Sambucol is a form of elderberry syrup that is widely available in health food stores, and it is often used for colds and sore throats as well as for the flu.

Herbs may also be helpful for pregnant women who suffer from allergies. A combination of nettle, eyebright, and yerba santa tinctures may give relief from the runny nose and weepy eyes that characterize some allergic reactions. Yerba manza and grindelia tinctures may relieve the sinus and nasal congestion that characterizes other allergies.

A number of herbs are safe for use by pregnant women while others are contraindicated. It is important for pregnant women to tell their obstetrical caretaker if they are using herbs. If you are under the care of an herbologist, let him or her know that you are pregnant so that they can modify your treatments, if necessary, and develop others.

CHAPTER SEVEN

Exercise during Pregnancy

It was once widely believed that pregnant women should rest as much as possible, stay in bed whenever possible, and avoid exercise and sex. Those days are long gone. Today's pregnant woman is likely to exercise at a health club, jog, and/or participate in sports on a regular basis. This can be good for the mother because many of the pains of pregnancy— back pain, hip soreness, and leg cramps—are due to the weight gain and decreased muscle strength of pregnancy. These might be avoided through proper conditioning and exercise.

In order to understand how exercise affects the fetus, let's explore what happens to the mother and her fetus when she exercises.

When a woman is pregnant, her body changes in ways that facilitate nourishing her baby. This means that more and more of her blood is sent to the uterus, placenta, and fetus as the pregnancy progresses. By the end of the twenty-eighth week of pregnancy, the blood supply to her uterus has increased ten times. By the end of the pregnancy, it has increased almost thirty times. This is because the baby needs more and more oxygen and nutrients as it grows, and it can only get these from the mother.

When a woman exercises, the skeletal muscles in her arms and legs need more blood and oxygen to nourish the parts that are working over-time. Since there is only so much blood in the body, the body must channel more blood to the skeletal muscles and less to internal organs like the stomach and uterus. When a woman exercises strenuously, the body has a conflict of interests—should it feed oxygen to the moving muscles or take care of the baby?

When the mother and baby are both healthy, fetuses get enough oxygen in spite of mild to moderate exercise on the mother's part. This is because a woman breathes faster and her heart beats faster when she exercises. This results in her getting more oxygen, which, in turn, circulates through both her and the baby. Thus, we don't believe that mild to moderate exercise causes fetal harm during a normal pregnancy. Fetuses do get heart decelerations during peak maternal exercise, but they don't translate into problems for the baby.

How much exercise is good for the fetus? We have found that the benefits of exercise during pregnancy are primarily for the mother, not for the fetus. If a woman exercised regularly before she got pregnant, she can do up to forty-five minutes of moderate exercise as often as she did before getting pregnant. Moderate exercise in pregnancy can be defined as activity that does not cause more than 120 heartbeats per minute. The heart rate should not stay there for more than twenty or thirty minutes.

A second aspect of concern about exercising during pregnancy is overheating. When someone exercises strenuously, the body's temperature increases, the blood vessels of the skin widen as they carry more blood, and the person perspires in order to cool off. As long as the mother does only mild to moderate exercise, she is able to cool off enough to prevent fetal overheating. Remember, the normal body temperature of the mother is over 98 degrees Fahrenheit, and the baby is usually slightly warmer.

Pregnant women also need to be concerned with dehydration. Dehydration can lead to uterine cramps and contractions and, in some cases, preterm labor. This makes it essential to drink enough water before, during, and after exercise, especially during the summer, to prevent ill effects of dehydration on the developing fetus.

The following guidelines on specific forms of exercise are for women with low-risk pregnancies. Women with uterine bleeding, who are at risk for preterm labor, who are pregnant with more than one fetus, or who have other high-risk factors are usually advised to avoid exercise during pregnancy. If a woman spotted during her first trimester, exercise is usually okay once she has stopped spotting for a week. Pregnant women should generally not undertake new forms of exercise. They should also discuss with their caretaker at an office visit if they need to modify their usual exercise routine.

Aerobic Exercise

Many health clubs offer aerobic exercise classes. It is generally safe for pregnant women to do aerobic exercise; however, like any type of weight-bearing activity, it may cause overheating or injury to the mother. If the jostling involved in any kind of exercise feels uncomfortable to the pregnant woman, she should stop. This is why pregnant women should take special aerobic classes that are geared for them and which are given by a qualified, experienced instructor.

Pregnant women need to be especially careful if they lift weights. Their bodies make a hormone called relaxin that relaxes the body's joints. Strained joints may be injured more easily during pregnancy. Also, heavy lifting more than fifteen times a day has been found to increase the risk of preterm labor, and heavy lifting along with strenuous work may result in low-birth-weight babies.

Once a woman is at least twenty weeks pregnant, she should avoid lying flat on her back because it can reduce blood flow to the baby. Any exercises that are normally done lying flat on one's back need to be modified.

Many doctors also discourage pregnant women from doing abdominal exercises, as they may predispose those muscles to separate permanently. When that happens, a woman will not be able to regain her previously flat abdomen.

Bicycling

Bicycling can be a good form of aerobic exercise during pregnancy, provided the woman can balance well enough to avoid injury. Since most pregnant women cannot do this by their fifth or sixth month, a stationary bicycle with a fan, or in an air-conditioned room, can be a good alternative. An added advantage of this type of exercise is that it is not weight-bearing, making it desirable for pregnant women.

Bowling

Bowling is generally okay as long as a woman does not strain her muscles.

High-Altitude Activities

Many people who vacation, hike, or exercise at high altitudes (above seven or eight thousand feet) get altitude sickness. Its symptoms are fatigue, headache, nausea, and getting "winded" quickly. This is due to the lack of oxygen at higher altitudes. A pregnant woman who exercises at these altitudes may not be able to get enough oxygen and should therefore avoid strenuous exercise in these environments. If she experiences altitude sickness, resting and staying well hydrated usually ameliorate the condition.

Hiking or Jogging and Lyme Disease

Women who hike or jog near wooded areas, especially in the northeastern part of the United States, are at risk for getting Lyme disease. Lyme disease is caused by a spirochete called *Borrelia burgdorferia*. People may get the disease when they are bitten by infected, immature deer ticks (*Ixodis dammini*). These ticks are most common in the late summer and early fall, in areas with bushes and tall grass.

After a person is bitten by an infected tick, Lyme disease can get into the bloodstream. It may go from there to the rest of the body, where it causes inflammation. The symptoms of Lyme disease are similar to those of the flu, including runny nose, general malaise, and headaches. However, unlike the flu, a rash lasting for a few days surrounds the area of the tick bite. Some weeks later, patients may get arthritis or pain in the large joints, especially in the knee or shoulder.

If left untreated, 20 percent of people with Lyme disease will get neurological problems such as Bell's palsy and aseptic meningitis. The disease may also inflame the heart muscle and cause chest pain and rapid heartbeat (palpitations).

Lyme disease is easy to misdiagnose. More than half of the people who are diagnosed did not know they were bitten by a tick. Some people who are infected may dismiss the rash as a mosquito or insect bite and think they got the flu. When joggers or athletes get joint pain, their pain may be misattributed to the running or athletic activity. The immunological tests for the disease (ELISA and indirect fluorescent antibody testing) often do not pick up Lyme disease when they are done in the early stages of the disease.

The spirochete that causes Lyme disease can affect the fetus if it crosses the placenta and enters the fetal compartment. When the Center for Disease Control studied pregnant women who had Lyme disease, none of their babies showed problems that could be directly linked to Lyme disease. When the mothers were treated for the disease, no long-term complications were noted in their babies.

Some medical literature once speculated that the spirochete causing Lyme disease may cause fetal death and miscarriage, but larger studies have not shown this to be true.

Pregnant women should avoid areas where they can get Lyme disease. Alternatively, if they walk or jog in tick-prone areas in the summer and early fall they should wear protective clothing that includes long-sleeved shirts and long pants or knee-high socks. If a woman gets the disease and it is in its early stages, most experts recommend that she get oral penicillin for ten to twelve days. If the disease is in the later stages, intravenous penicillin is usually recommended (provided, of course, that she is not allergic to penicillin; in such cases an alternative antibiotic is taken). Ingesting penicillin is not associated with any fetal abnormalities.

Diane was a forty-one-year-old teacher from upstate New York. When she was six weeks pregnant, she came to her obstetrician for her first visit. She told the doctor that she had a mild headache and a swollen and painful right knee. She assumed those were due to a twisted muscle caused by her daily jogging in wooded areas. The doctor advised her to stop jogging until her knee felt better, and told her to take Tylenol for the pain.

She returned to the doctor five days later because she discovered a rash on her right shoulder. At this point, the doctor had her tested for Lyme disease, and the test was positive. She was given oral antibiotics for ten days, during which time she resumed jogging, albeit wearing a long-sleeved shirt and lightweight pants. She eventually gave birth to a full-term, healthy baby girl. The baby was tested for Lyme disease and did not have it. The baby is three years old now and developing normally.

Jogging

Research has shown that women who jog between one and two and a half miles a day during pregnancy suffer no ill effects, nor do their babies. Women who are used to jogging longer distances should not jog more than two to two and a half miles a day. While jogging, it is important to keep checking one's pulse periodically and make sure it stays under 120 beats per minute. This is because the baby's heart rate is directly related to the mother's. If the baby's heart rate goes above 180 beats per minute, it can potentially cause problems with the baby's heart.

Thus, women who jog regularly before they get pregnant may do so during pregnancy, as long as they jog moderately and avoid overexertion, overheating, and dehydration. They should also be careful during the last trimester when their balance is not as good and their muscles are weaker. We recommend that they choose a running surface that is comfortable and wear shoes with proper arch supports. In extreme conditions (heat, high humidity, or extreme cold) we suggest avoiding jogging; brisk walking is better.

Scuba Diving

Little research has been done on the effects of scuba diving on the fetus, but it is known that scuba diving causes nitrogen to build up in the blood. One can potentially get decompression sickness (the "bends") and decreased oxygen to the uterus, placenta, and fetus. Pregnant women should never scuba dive because of these potential dangers. If one has a yen to swim with fish or view coral while pregnant, try surface snorkeling instead in places that do not have rocks or coral close to the surface.

If you went scuba diving during the two weeks after conception and then discovered you were pregnant, you probably don't need to worry. Anecdotal reports from scuba instructors who dove until their pregnancies were confirmed have not shown any increased incidence of birth defects.

Swimming

Swimming is probably the best type of exercise during pregnancy because the body doesn't have to bear weight. Consequently, the joints are not stressed, and it is hard to get overheated in a pool or the ocean. Lap swimming allows a pregnant woman to get a good amount of aerobic exercise, and there is no established limit as to how long a pregnant woman can swim. She should stop whenever she feels tired, cold, and/or has difficulty breathing. The water should not be very cold or very hot, with a temperature of 75–82 degrees Fahrenheit being ideal.

Women often wonder if swimming can result in uterine infections. Many studies have tested this by dyeing the water in which a woman swims and seeing how much enters her vagina and/or uterus. The conclusion is that no water enters. Therefore, a woman can feel free to swim in swimming pools, lakes, rivers, and oceans, provided they are not contaminated in ways that would present a risk to anyone.

Tennis

Tennis, like many other athletic activities, requires a pregnant woman to frequently adjust to her shifting center of gravity. Some pregnant woman feel clumsier and they stumble and/or fall from time to time. If a woman was an avid tennis player before she got pregnant, there is no reason to stop, provided she exercises in moderation and compensates for her shift in balance. Competitive tennis is not recommended; playing doubles is a good choice.

Athletics to Avoid

The following types of physical activity should be avoided by pregnant women because of the high risk of injury: contact sports, volleyball, basketball, gymnastics, downhill skiing, horseback riding, ice skating, roller skating, Rollerblading, karate, boxing, kick-boxing, football, and soccer.

When choosing any form of exercise, women should remember that their bones and muscles soften toward the end of pregnancy. At those times it is easier to get injured even during "safe" forms of exercise than when a woman is not pregnant.

Jacuzzis

When a pregnant woman has had a stressful day, her back aches, she has just finished exercising, or she simply wants to relax, she may be tempted to slip into a hot jacuzzi and melt away the tension. This is a very bad idea, especially during the first trimester. If the jacuzzi is hotter than 96 degrees Fahrenheit, stay away. (The same holds true for hot baths.) Scientific reports have linked overheating in a jacuzzi during the first few weeks of pregnancy with the baby developing neural tube defects.

If you want to relax in hot water after exercising, take a hot shower for no more than five or ten minutes. When we are overheated, we normally cool down by perspiring. When the area surrounding the fetus is immersed in hot water, perspiring does not cool it down, and that area of the body can become as hot as the water surrounding it. This is why it's important not to overheat the baby by having the mother soak in a very hot tub or the like. Putting one's legs in a hot tub, or soaking in a very warm bath without immersing the abdomen, is fine.

Massage

Massage can be wonderful when it is done by a licensed massage therapist who knows how to work with pregnant women. It can reduce emotional stress and cause release of endorphins (those "feel-good" chemicals), reduce back, leg, and headache pain, and help with sciatica and ankle swelling. It improves circulation and can give temporary relief from the pain of varicose veins. Some women find that massage during labor helps them relax and feel more comfortable.

It is important that a pregnant woman in her fourth month and beyond lie on her side while she gets a massage, so that her weight doesn't compress the blood supply to her uterus. Unless it is desirable for a woman to go into labor, stimulating certain "abortion" points around the sacrum and calf which can initiate uterine contractions should also be avoided.

Working during Pregnancy

*T*oday, *most first-time mothers work outside the home. Whether or* not pregnancy should change their work life depends upon their general health, how the fetus is doing, what the women do at work, and what they are exposed to there.

Studies have shown that women with low-risk pregnancies, whose work is no more physically demanding than what they would do otherwise, can safely work until they go into labor. They can then resume work a few weeks after giving birth.

Some women develop problems such as edema, high blood pressure, or a dilated cervix. These conditions make it advisable to work less or not at all. Other women are already so physically challenged at work that doing the same job during pregnancy might be ill-advised or dangerous. These might include working long hours in the hot sun, jobs that require a lot of climbing or careful balancing, or prolonged standing. If a woman has an opportunity to get off her feet, she should use it.

There are also many potential environmental hazards at work that reduce the amount of oxygen that pregnant women can get. Smoke (cigarette and otherwise), exhaust fumes, sawdust, particulate matter, industrial solvents, metals such as lead and mercury, and bacteria and viruses in laboratories and hospitals can all harm pregnant women, and may necessitate switching jobs for a while.

Approximately 10 percent of birth defects are due to contaminants to which pregnant women are exposed at work. Women's work may expose them to toxic vapors or to toxic materials that are absorbed through their skin. They may inadvertently consume toxic products by eating with hands that are contaminated, or by putting hands or cigarettes that were contaminated into their mouths. Women who work in laboratories; chemical or industrial factories; dry cleaning institutions; nail salons; textile, glass, pottery, or electronic manufacturing; radiation departments; food and drink industries; and printing institutions are among those most at risk. So are those who work with paints, varnishes, and shellacs.

Pregnant women who were exposed to lots of automobile exhaust have been shown to have higher rates of miscarriage. Women who worked at jobs where they were exposed to vinyl chloride (found in plastics) had higher rates of miscarriage or babies with neural tube defects, chromosomal abnormalities, and newborn death. Obviously, people who can choose jobs where they avoid these substances, and who can travel on roads where they are not exposed to heavy air pollution, should do so.

Professional women who have stressful jobs, such as medical residents, law clerks, and delivery room nurses, have more complications during pregnancy, as do pregnant women who work long hours, who do heavy lifting, who stand for long periods, and so on. They should seriously consider modifying their work hours or conditions while pregnant.

The Civil Rights Act of 1964 states that employers with at least fifteen workers cannot refuse to hire someone because she is pregnant. Nor can they deny her credit for previous years, accrued retirement benefits, or seniority because she takes maternity leave. Pregnant women must be allowed to continue to work as long as they can do their job. If the company will not let her take sick leave, it may be discriminatory.

Pregnant or postpartum women must be treated the same as other employees who can't work for a short period of time. For example, if it is company policy that workers may do light work if they hurt their back, or get unpaid disability leave because they have medical problems, pregnant women are entitled to the same.

California, Hawaii, New Jersey, New York, Rhode Island, and Puerto Rico have temporary disability insurance. That is, they pay partial salaries when someone can't work due to a medical problem or pregnancy.

The Family and Medical Leave Act gives pregnant women up to twelve weeks of unpaid leave if a doctor attests that they can't work. Postpartum women are also entitled to six weeks' off if they have a vaginal delivery, and eight weeks off for a cesarean section. When women go back to work, they have the right to get the same job back, or one with the same pay and benefits.

Some pregnant women need to stop working because they require bed rest, while others need temporary reassignment because their job exposes them to toxins or hazardous working conditions. For example, a policewoman may not want to participate in firearms training because the noise may be harmful to the developing fetus. An airline baggage handler should not lift heavy suitcases and the like. A woman who works with heavy machinery might be transferred to office work until she gives birth.

Pregnant women who need to prove disability in order to get payments or reassignment may get forms from their employer. Women need to bring these to their doctor's office where the forms will be completed truthfully and sent back to the employer. Doctors will not create a disability when there is none.

Women who think they were discriminated against because of their pregnancy may file charges with the U.S. Equal Employment Opportunity Commissioner (1-800-669-EEOC), even if they no longer work for the employer. They may also contact the Women's Bureau of the U.S. Department of Labor (1-800-827-5335).

CHAPTER NINE

Travel during Pregnancy

W omen today travel more than ever before, for both business and pleasure. While some women make travel plans knowing they are pregnant, half of the pregnancies that occur are unplanned. This means that many women will have purchased tickets and made travel plans without taking into consideration that they might be expecting when they go away.

Ideally, pregnant women should not travel to places where they can't get good obstetrical care in an emergency. Pregnancy is challenging enough for some women that they don't want to find themselves unexpectedly ill, needing to be airlifted somewhere, or traveling on unpaved roads for hours before they can be evaluated or treated. When we plan trips, we like to assume that they will go more or less as planned. Frequent travelers learn from experience that that may not be a good assumption.

Air Travel

Air travel today is one of the safest modes of transportation for most people, but is it safe for the fetus? The first question to address is what happens to the fetus when the mother goes from ground level to thousands of feet up in the air.

Most commercial airlines today have pressurized cabins, although very small commuter planes may not. It is safe for the fetus when pregnant women travel in pressurized cabins.

Cabin pressure is rarely an issue for domestic travel, but unpressurized cabins can be encountered when traveling short distances in Alaska, when island hopping, or in a foreign country. If you plan to travel under these circumstances, check with the air carrier and find out if the cabin is pressurized.

A second problem that occurs when people fly is the greater exposure to viruses and bacteria that can make them sick. Sitting in an enclosed cabin with recirculated air means passengers have a greater than normal chance of breathing in airborne "bugs." If one travels at a time of year when people tend to be sick, such as fall or winter, it is easy for a pregnant woman to be exposed to viruses or bacteria. If there are a number of children on the flight, or a sick one nearby, she might also have a greater chance of being exposed to childhood illnesses for which she is not protected. The longer the flight, the greater the chance of being infected. Some women might therefore prefer not to fly at certain times of the year, or to destinations that have crowded flights with lots of children onboard.

In addition, airline air is not humidified. This, combined with the reduced air pressure that normally occurs on flights, makes it necessary to drink extra fluid in order to stay hydrated. Some pregnant women carry a water bottle with them for convenience when they fly.

As we mention elsewhere in this book, dehydration can result in preterm labor. It is very important to drink a lot of nonalcoholic, noncaffeinated beverages while flying. Alcohol and caffeine enhance dehydration.

People who travel on airlines tend to sit still for long periods of time. Since pregnant women have a greater likelihood of getting blood clots in their legs, it is recommended that they not cross their legs when sitting, and they should get up and walk for a few minutes every one to three hours. This increases circulation in their legs and helps keep blood going to the fetus. This is especially important when the pregnancy is beyond the fourth month. If you drink enough fluid, you will probably find yourself doing this anyway as you go back and forth to the restroom.

Some doctors recommend that pregnant women take a baby aspirin before going on a long flight, in order to improve their blood circulation.

When Pregnant Women Can't Fly

Every airline has its own policy about when pregnant women can't travel. Most airlines in the United States allow women to travel to international destinations until at least thirty days before their due date, and to domestic cities until a week to thirty days before their due date. Foreign countries have varying guidelines about when pregnant women can fly. If you plan to travel during your last trimester, be sure to call each airline you will use ahead of time and find out what their policies are for domestic and international travel. If you are very big or far along, it is also a good idea to carry a note from your practitioner saying that it is safe for you to fly.

We do not recommend that women with uncomplicated pregnancies fly anywhere during their eighth or ninth month unless it is absolutely necessary. This is because a woman could always go into labor earlier than expected.

Remember that short flights can sometimes end up being much longer. If that happens and you need obstetrical attention, there are a few things that you can do. First, the airline attendants can alert any doctors that happen to be onboard, or they can arrange for a doctor or ambulance to meet the plane at the destination. Also, cell phones and airphones allow women to call their usual caretaker from almost anywhere today.

Boat Travel

One of the main practical concerns about boat travel during pregnancy is what to do for seasickness. Since this can ruin a vacation, it's often a good idea to cancel one's travel plans if the boat may travel in waters that are not calm.

If one is set on taking a cruise, what can pregnant women safely do to combat seasickness?

Scopolamine patches, the most common remedy, are not considered safe for pregnant women to use. Some people find that taking an extract (tincture) of American ginger, or drinking some grated fresh ginger mixed with water, is effective. Other people swear by accupressure bracelets that alleviate nausea by putting pressure on two points near the wrist. If all else fails, try to stay upright and fix your gaze on the horizon in a place that you can get fresh air.

Before a pregnant woman plans a boat trip, we recommend asking the boat operator what kind of weather and sea conditions are likely at that time of year and what their cancellation policy is. Remember, the boat company is interested in making money and will not usually cancel an outing because passengers will feel queasy. Their standards regarding reasonable sea weather might be quite different from those of the passengers.

Even if the cruise or boat trip has already been paid for, a pregnant woman should try to find out before leaving what kind of weather and sea conditions are expected. Having morning sickness is bad enough. Being pitched to and fro for hours or days while having morning sickness can be worth avoiding at almost any cost, even if it means losing the entire purchase price of your trip.

A final note about boat travel: Ships have various methods by which passengers can get into and out of the boat. Some require climbing up or down steep ladders on the side of the ship, then getting into dinghies that ferry passengers to shore. Others have ramps with much firmer footing. If a woman is far along in her pregnancy, she might not be comfortable traveling on boats or cruises that use dinghies and side ladders. Find out how your intended cruise line transfers passengers from ship to shore before booking.

Automobile Travel

While domestic car travel seems to present few hazards to the pregnant woman, road conditions that we take for granted in the United States might be almost unheard-of in other parts of the world. For example, some Caribbean countries with beautiful beaches and tropical climates have roads with potholes big enough to take off a car axle. Their automobile tracks are made from mud and rocks instead of asphalt; others are made of sand with poor traction. The maximum speed that one can safely go in some of these places is 15 mph. Even at such slow speeds, a pregnant woman will have her belly bounced around in unnerving ways. That lovely little park or historic site that the brochure says is worth visiting may be the last place a pregnant woman will want to go. Call an automobile association for details about road conditions in places that are off the beaten track or in foreign countries.

This is also worth doing for trips in the United States, especially in winter. Some roads are passable only if you have four-wheel-drive. Roads in Western mountain areas are routinely closed due to avalanches. Some national parks have snow, ice, and extreme weather conditions even during the late spring or early summer. Be prepared with suitable clothes, extra water and food, and a cell phone. Don't find yourself stranded in places you don't want to be without adequate warmth, food, and water.

When pregnant women drive, they should recline against the back-rest, and use a lower back support if the seat is deep. Wear a safety belt with the lap part under the belly, across the upper thigh.

Protection against Diseases

Before traveling to a foreign country, find out what diseases are prevalent there. One of the best sources of information for this is the Centers for Disease Control in Atlanta, Georgia. They also have a website (www.cdc.gov) that tells what diseases are prevalent in a specific locale, and what vaccinations are recommended before traveling there. One can also contact a particular country's embassy or travel center in the United States to get more information. Most of these are located in New York City or Washington, D.C.

See pages 161–167 on preventing infections and for a discussion of common diseases such as malaria or hepatitis that a woman may encounter while traveling.

If a trip to game parks in places like South Africa has already been set up, and a pregnant woman is intent on going, she should take certain precautions. While many game parks do have malaria during the wet season, they may be malaria-free during the dry season. It may also be easier to see game at that time because they cluster closer to watering holes. Game parks that are in higher and drier areas tend to be malaria-free year-round, and they also abound with wildlife. Contact the individual game lodges and parks for more information.

Availability of Medical Care and Medication

Nothing can spoil a vacation or business trip more quickly than a medical crisis. Pregnant women may not be concerned about the presence of adequate medical facilities at their destination unless an emergency develops.

Despite recent changes in American health care, we are still spoiled by the relative availability of medical care and drugs. We don't think twice about what to do if we develop strep throat and need antibiotics the same day, or if we have a medical problem and need to see a doctor within twenty-four hours. This is often not the case when traveling, especially outside the United States.

Remember that accidents happen. Take a duplicate set of medications, prescriptions, syringes if necessary, and your medical history when you travel. Always make sure to keep one set with your hand luggage when you travel on airplanes. Do a little research in advance about what resources are available should you have a medical or obstetrical problem. Make sure that you have a way of contacting your health care professional back home if you need to. Get the names and phone numbers of a nearby medical center and doctor (the manager of the hotel may be able to tell you whom they use when necessary), and know what hours someone is on call. You might want to postpone a trip until after you give birth if the medical resources of the place you want to go are very limited.

Attitudes about Pregnant Women

One of the least discussed aspects of travel is the attitude people in various places have about pregnant women. Americans take for granted that pregnant women get extra consideration, such as having someone give away a seat on a crowded bus or subway, or giving help with a heavy door when she is carrying heavy things. Unfortunately, some people in other countries do not take kindly to pregnant women being seen in public and do not give them any courtesies.

In some Muslim countries, for example, pregnant women do not go out in public. It is considered almost promiscuous for a woman who is obviously expecting to walk about in public view. One of our pregnant patients went to the market in Yemen by herself in the 1990s. Despite her modest attire, she was beaten for walking in a public place. Another pregnant woman reported an untoward series of experiences when she went to a different Muslim country in her third trimester.

Debbie and her husband loved history, nature, and walking. They thought that they could combine all these interests by going to Turkey to see the archeological ruins, the souks, museums, palaces, and beaches. Much to their horror, the local children and women everywhere crowded around Debbie's protruding belly, pointing, mocking, and staring. It was not until the end of the trip that they realized that they never saw another pregnant woman during their stay. When they asked an English-speaking guide if that was coincidental, he confirmed that once a pregnant woman "shows," she usually stays sequestered until after she gives birth.

In some cities, pregnant women are also easy targets for pickpockets and muggers. If you are planning a trip to a place that has street crime, such as some cities in South America or Eastern Europe, make sure to wear a money belt or conceal your money next to your body. Be smart about not wearing jewelry, handbags, or a nice watch.

While learning about a foreign country's geography, culture, food, and languages will enhance your visit, we recommend learning about their attitudes toward pregnant women before you go.

Pregnant women should also keep in mind that their participation at certain vacation attractions may be restricted, both in the United States and elsewhere. For example, amusement and theme parks such as Disney World, Astroworld, and the like prohibit (with good reason) pregnant women from going on certain rides. You might want to go elsewhere when you are pregnant.

One last anecdote will suffice to illustrate the importance of calling ahead to unusual vacation spots and inquiring if there are any restrictions on pregnant women's participation.

Mary and her husband both loved swimming and underwater sea life, so they planned a vacation that included an opportunity to swim with dolphins. They were most excited about doing this for the first time. Since Mary was just ending her third month of pregnancy, she did not think there was any risk in swimming with these delightful animals.

Much to her surprise, the guide who gave the mandatory orientation said that their establishment would not allow pregnant women to swim with the dolphins. Dolphins have excellent sonar and can see that a woman is pregnant, just as a doctor sees the fetus on a sonogram. Dolphins are very solicitous of pregnant women, just as they are of pregnant dolphins, and they tend to rally around pregnant women just as they do their own. While the idea of having a "support group" of several female dolphins may sound like fun, the reality of being surrounded (and bumped) by half a dozen three- to four-hundred pound swimming mammals may not be. When they bump into the woman they could possibly harm her, despite their protective intentions.

In summary, if you want to travel while pregnant, be well prepared, well informed, and expect the unexpected.

CHAPTER TEN

Multiple Pregnancies

*J*ust *a few decades ago, it was rare for women to have multiple gesta-*tions, or pregnancies with more than one fetus. Twins occurred once in ninety births, triplets only once in a thousand. Since the advent of assisted fertility, though, there has been an explosion of multiples such that even octuplets are possible. While in the days of baby boomers a school might have one or two sets of twins—who were considered objects of curiosity—some schools today have many, along with a sprinkling of triplets. With one out of five or six couples having infertility problems, we can imagine the prevalence of multiple pregnancies for some time to come.

While multiple pregnancies can be uneventful, they are much more likely than singleton births to have problems. The most common problems are preterm birth and low birth weight, where the baby is born before thirty-seven weeks and weighs less than five and a half pounds. Full-term babies are born between thirty-seven and forty-two weeks, while the average twin is born at thirty-five to thirty-six weeks, and the average triplet or quad is born far earlier.

While some twins are born full-term, others are born so early that they die or bear the consequences of prematurity forever. About 6 percent of twins weigh less than 2.2 pounds when they are born.

We don't know why women with multiple pregnancies tend to go into labor early but it seems that labor starts as soon as the uterus is filled to a certain capacity. Obviously, the space is taken up much more quickly when there is more than one fetus.

The greater chance that women with multiple fetuses will go into preterm labor makes it crucial for them to rest as much as possible. If a woman's first pregnancy is with twins, she may be advised to rest in bed during the day and stop working at as early as twenty-six weeks. Some, though, will continue their daily routine under close supervision until they give birth.

Women with multiple fetuses need to know the sometimes subtle signs and symptoms of premature labor. They need to contact their caretaker if they feel abdominal pain or tightening, cramping, or back pain, or if they get markedly increased vaginal mucus or any bloody discharge.

Back in the 1980s and 1990s, women with multiple pregnancies routinely monitored their contractions twice a day using home devices. The tape was transmitted to specially trained nurses at a central station. They let the doctors know if a woman had an unacceptable pattern of contractions. The woman could then be treated or sent to the hospital, as necessary. Most studies have failed to show that home monitoring provides any real advantages for low-risk women, so this expensive service is now reserved only for special circumstances, such as for women who cannot feel contractions that open up her cervix.

Premature rupture of membranes is also more common in multiple pregnancies. This is discussed further in the chapter on premature birth. (See page 218.)

Besides prematurity, mothers of multiples are much more likely to get toxemia, diabetes, stunted fetal growth, or bleeding problems such as placenta previa. That is why women carrying twins are usually seen by their caretaker every two to three weeks until the third trimester, and every week or two subsequently. They get ultrasounds every month until the last month, at which time they are done every week. Women expecting triplets or more see their caretakers for additional visits. Women expecting multiples are also more likely than singleton mothers to be hospitalized when they have worrisome problems such as rising blood pressure.

Discordance

One problem unique to multiples is discordancy, when one twin weighs at least 20–25 percent less than the other. This can be seen on serial ultrasounds. For example, if one twin weighs 5.5 pounds and the other weighs 4.5 pounds, they are discordant. This may be due to normal variation between two babies, but it can also reflect the placenta's inability to deliver enough nutrients to one fetus.

Identical twins, who develop from one fertilized egg that then splits into two zygotes, can also have problems from sharing the same blood supply. This is called twin-to-twin transfusion syndrome (or "stuck twin syndrome"). It causes one twin to get more blood than the other. The former twin is larger, has a higher (often too high) blood count, and more amniotic fluid (often too much) around it. Meanwhile, the latter twin is small, anemic, pale, and has little amniotic fluid around it. The term "stuck twin" describes the fact that this twin appears to be stuck against the wall of the uterus.

The excess fluid around the larger twin dooms this pregnancy unless as much as several quarts of fluid are drawn away at a time. This needs to be repeated as necessary. This is done by using a needle and syringe under sonographic guidance, similar to an amniocentesis.

A more aggressive way of treating this is to use a laser to cut a hole between the two babies' sacs so that the fluid can redistribute itself more evenly.

These pregnancies need to be watched closely, and they are usually delivered early, often by cesarean section.

In 1 percent of twin pregnancies, identical twins share the same sac, without the partition that usually separates them and their umbilical cords. Their umbilical cords may intertwine, potentially killing one or both babies. Women with monoamniotic twins are watched closely and hospitalized early. They usually get nonstress tests twice a day, and sonograms two to three times a week. Some obstetricians even prescribe continuous fetal monitoring for weeks. These women are then delivered by cesarean section long before they are due.

Pregnancy Reduction

Infertility treatments have resulted in pregnancies of three or more fetuses, where extreme prematurity and death occur frequently. For example, for every set of surviving sextuplets, probably ten sets have disabilities or die. Since some of these mothers are unlikely to have another successful pregnancy, doctors have devised a way to sacrifice one or more fetuses in an attempt to safeguard the lives of the others. Otherwise all or most of the fetuses are likely to die. This procedure may be religiously or personally objectionable to some women.

Congenital Defects

Twins have more congenital abnormalities than singletons do. Identical twins have more structural deformities, while fraternal twins have twice as many chromosomal or genetic defects. This is because each twin has its own chance of having a defect. These are added together since there are two babies. Thus, a forty-year-old woman has almost a 1 percent chance of having a single baby with Down syndrome. If she is pregnant with fraternal twins, the risk is 2 percent, or one chance in fifty.

This can present heart-rending choices to women about whether they should have an amniocentesis. If so, should they abort one twin if it has a major anomaly? They must take into account the fact that aborting one fetus will increase the chance that the surviving fetus will be delivered prematurely, with all the attendant problems.

Multiple Births

Delivering multiple babies can be complex, so some doctors automatically deliver twins by cesarean section. However, if twins are both head-down, and aren't monoamniotic or high risk because of twin-to-twin transfusion syndrome or some other problem, a vaginal delivery can be done safely and should be tried.

Once the first twin is delivered vaginally, it can take up to an hour for the second twin to be born. During this time, the second baby's heartbeat should be monitored because several problems may occur. First, his placenta may separate (abrupt) from the uterine wall. Second, since his head is probably not low, his umbilical cord has a greater chance of slipping down (prolapsing) in front of him into the vagina. Since cord prolapse is much more common if the second twin's water is broken, most obstetricians will not break the second bag of water until the baby's head is well down into the pelvis. Meanwhile, they give the mother intravenous Pitocin to increase the power of the contractions that will quickly push out that twin.

When the second twin is breech (head-up) or transverse (sideways), many practitioners do a cesarean section, especially if this is the mother's first birth. Other practitioners will attempt a vaginal delivery. But cesarean sections are preferred by most doctors if the second twin is breech and much larger than the first, or if the twins are premature. Heads of "preemies" are much larger than their bodies, and they are more delicate than full-term babies. Thus, a breech preemie's feet might deliver easily through a vagina while the head gets stuck in the pelvis.

Few doctors will vaginally deliver total breech singleton babies today, unless the woman has had many prior deliveries. They are worried that the head might get stuck in the pelvis after the rest of the baby delivers.

On the other hand, many practitioners feel that a vaginal delivery is easier when there are twins, the second of whom is breech. They use the baby's feet as a handle to pull him out of the uterus through a vagina that was just opened up by the first baby. (This is called a total breech presentation.)

If a second twin is transverse, it will often become breech or head-down once the first twin is delivered, especially if a practitioner pushes on the uterus in a way that guides the baby into a better position. If the second twin stays transverse, its feet cannot be used to pull it into a breech position, and it must be delivered by cesarean section.

There are times when the first twin was delivered vaginally, yet the second one must be delivered by cesarean section. This might occur if the second twin is stuck in a transverse position, his cord is prolapsing down, or his placenta is tearing away from the uterus.

When there are three or more babies in a pregnancy, they are almost invariably delivered by cesarean section. While a rare practitioner will attempt vaginal delivery of triplets, a cesarean section makes for an easy and gentle delivery, with a uterus that is easy to cut and sew back together.

Getting Support

While there is a collective sigh of relief when multiple babies are delivered and all has gone well, this is only the beginning for the parents. The mother will have to recuperate physically while being under tremendous stress from the continual demands of her new family. The babies may seem to need around-the-clock feeding, burping, clothing, and diaper-changing. It is easy for the mother to feel that she is ill equipped and too exhausted for the tasks at hand.

Many couples find the experience overwhelming, but it is important to remember that things do get easier over time. It is critical to try to get as much extra help, emotional support, and encouragement as possible. Those who have the financial wherewithal should hire a baby nurse who is experienced in taking care of multiples for the first few weeks. Family and friends can be invaluable doing basic chores such as bottle-feeding, cooking, cleaning, laundry, and taking care of other children.

There are several support groups and national organizations for parents of multiples such as Mothers of Super Twins (most.org) and the Triplet Connection. These not only give emotional support and child-rearing information, they also give practical ideas about where to buy baby furnishings or get items free of charge. Learn about these organizations and peruse their magazines long before the babies are due to get a head start. Remember, eventually things will get much easier.

PART II

If Problems Arise

CHAPTER ELEVEN

Will My Baby Be Normal?

One of the first questions that expectant parents ask after discovering they are pregnant is, "Will my baby be normal?" Although there are no guarantees that a baby will be healthy, a few tests can reassure the majority of women that they are not likely to have a baby with major birth defects. Before we discuss these tests, it is important to have a basic understanding of what birth defects are and how they occur.

Birth Defects

About 2–3 percent of babies are born with a major birth defect, half of which are immediately obvious. These fall into four possible types of defects: chromosomal anomalies, single-gene disorders, multifactorial inheritance, and teratogenic disorders.

Body cells contain chromosomes that tell the cell what to do. When cells reproduce, the chromosomes cause that cell's traits to be programmed into new cells. Thus, hair cells make new hair cells instead of skin cells, and mucous membrane cells make more of the same instead of brain cells, and so on. Each chromosome contains many genes, each of which gives specific information to the cell about what it needs to do. There are genes that control eye color, blood type, the shape of the ears,

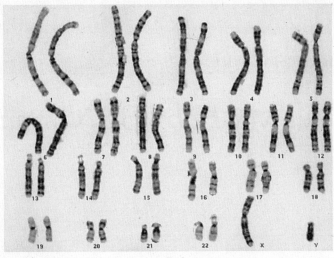

Fig. 2

hair color, and so on. In addition, a typical person has five to eight genes that predispose the person to getting specific diseases.

The recently completed genome project will allow us to know the detailed order of human genes, almost like reading a book about the subject. Hopefully, this will soon help scientists predict and treat genetic disorders.

People have twenty-two pairs of regular chromosomes and one pair of sex chromosomes (see fig. 2). When an egg is fertilized, each parent contributes its chromosomes. The mother's egg automatically contributes an X chromosome. Some sperm have an X chromosome, while others have a Y. If the father's sperm contained an X chromosome, the baby will be a girl. If it had a Y chromosome, the baby will be a boy.

Chromosomal Anomalies

Girls are born with all of the eggs they will ever have (up to four hundred thousand), although only one is released every month during the reproductive years. As women get older, their eggs age with them, unlike a man's sperm, which are made new on an ongoing basis. Older eggs are more likely to make chromosomal errors, so the chances of having chromosomal anomalies such as Down syndrome and trisomy 18 increase with the mother's age. Older fathers do not have much more risk of fathering children with chromosomal anomalies than younger men do.

Sometimes, when fertilization occurs, a future embryo gets the wrong number of chromosomes. This is known as a chromosomal anomaly. For example, a fetus might get an extra chromosome, as happens with Down syndrome. Such babies have trisomy 21, or an extra 21st chromosome. Babies with Down syndrome have varying degrees of mental retardation and physical defects. These include a flattened face, a large, protruding tongue, and poor muscle tone. Many also have heart and gastrointestinal defects. Due to advances in pediatric surgery, special education, and nutrition for such children, having a child with Down today is not the same as it was years ago. The average life expectancy of someone with Down is now around fifty-five years, and their quality of life is often quite good. Many of the physical problems that were assumed to be inevitable can now be ameliorated by giving Down children specific nutritional supplements starting from birth.

About one in eight hundred babies is born with Down syndrome. Women who already have a child with Down, or who are thirty-five or older, are more likely than other women to have a child with Down, as can be seen from the table on page 112.

Trisomy 18 occurs when a baby gets an extra eighteenth chromosome, causing profound mental retardation and severe, multiple physical defects. This disease is far less common than Down syndrome, and such babies usually die during the first year of life.

Some chromosomal defects are caused by the chromosome breaking. One of the most common causes of mental retardation in American males is fragile X syndrome, where the X chromosome breaks at a fragile point. Because males have only one X chromosome and females have two X's, a break there usually affects only males. Females may "carry" this trait in their eggs and pass it to their male offspring, but they aren't usually affected themselves. If there is a family history of mental retardation, especially in males, fragile X screening can be considered. Unless

Estimated Chance That a Baby Will Have Down Syndrome Based on the Mother's Age

Age	Chance of Having a Baby with Down Syndrome	Age	Chance of Having a Baby with Down Syndrome
20	1 in 1,528	33	1 in 574
21	1 in 1,507	34	1 in 474
22	1 in 1,481	35	1 in 384
23	1 in 1,447	36	1 in 307
24	1 in 1,404	37	1 in 242
25	1 in 1,351	38	1 in 189
26	1 in 1,286	39	1 in 146
27	1 in 1,208	40	1 in 112
28	1 in 1,119	41	1 in 85
29	1 in 1,018	42	1 in 65
30	1 in 909	43	1 in 49
31	1 in 796	44	1 in 37
32	1 in 683	45	1 in 28

special stains of amniocentesis fluid are done, the defective arms of a fragile X chromosome cannot be seen when a regular amniocentesis is done.

Single-Gene Disorders

Sickle-cell anemia, Tay-Sachs, cystic fibrosis, Von Willebrand's disease, and hemophilia are all single-gene disorders. These defects occur because a specific gene is abnormal. Traits that need the problematic gene to be contributed from both parents are known as recessive, and those that can be inherited from only one parent are known as dominant. For example, Tay-Sachs, a recessive genetic trait common among Ashkenazic Jews, requires both parents to contribute the faulty gene for a baby to be affected. A parent who has a specific gene is known as a carrier. If the other parent is not a carrier, recessive traits are not passed on to offspring, but dominant traits might be.

If both parents carry the Tay-Sachs gene, for example, each has a normal gene and an abnormal one. There is a 50 percent chance that each parent will give the baby a normal gene, and a 50 percent chance that each will give an abnormal one. A quick calculation shows that a baby will have a 25 percent chance of getting a Tay-Sachs gene from each parent, and thereby get the disease. There is a 50 percent chance that the child will be a carrier but not have the disease, and a 25 percent chance that a baby will not be a carrier and will not have the disease.

Thus, when a disease is transmitted through recessive genes, there is a 25 percent chance of a child getting the disease if both parents are carriers, and virtually no chance of getting the disease if only one parent is a carrier. It is now understandable why a person could be a carrier for a genetic disorder without anyone else in the family having it. If another carrier of the recessive gene marries into one's family, it can unmask the disease.

The most common problematic recessive gene among whites is cystic fibrosis. Children born with cystic fibrosis have serious problems in their lungs and bowels, and the disease may be fatal, usually in early adulthood. The severity of cystic fibrosis varies from person to person. Some need minimal respiratory care and live normal lives, while others may die despite having lung transplants.

Sickle-cell anemia is the most common serious recessive gene among blacks, with one in ten being a carrier. About one in four hundred black children who are conceived has the disease. Its symptoms are low blood counts and painful crises. People with this form of anemia often need pain control and blood transfusions.

Couples can be screened via simple blood tests before they get married to see if they carry any genes for lethal or serious disorders. Some couples decide not to marry when they discover they are both carriers of a serious genetic disorder. Married couples can get screened, then see a genetic counselor before having children if they both carry a serious disease. Some such couples will decide to adopt, or use donor eggs or sperm to achieve a pregnancy.

Multifactorial Inheritance

These disorders are inherited via more than one gene. Most abnormal babies who don't have a chromosomal anomaly or single-gene disorder have a multifactorially inherited disease. These include neural tube defects (see page 139), heart disease, and club foot. These are inherited in a very complex way such that the chances of having a second child if a prior one already had a disorder is about 2–5 percent. The risk is higher if one already had two or more affected children.

Teratogenic Disorders

These are birth defects caused by substances to which the mother is exposed during pregnancy. For example, 2–5 percent of pregnant women who take the anti-seizure medication valproic acid have babies with neural tube defects, and pregnant women who take Coumadin give birth to babies with birth defects. However, as the majority of women stop taking Coumadin when they become pregnant, this effect is rarely seen today. (Teratogens are discussed in chapter 12.) Women who had chemotherapy with dactinomycin prior to getting pregnant have an increased rate of babies with heart defects, although having other forms of chemotherapy prior to getting pregnant has not been related to an increased rate of babies with chromosomal anomalies.

CHAPTER TWELVE

Will It Harm the Baby?

*A*ll *women would like to have a healthy baby, and 97–98 percent of* babies are born without major birth defects. Nevertheless, women need to know what kinds of substances and circumstances can potentially harm their baby. Three types of women can potentially have more problems than others, so we recommend that they consult a practitioner or genetics counselor before becoming pregnant. They are: women who use prescription medications, alcohol, or recreational drugs; women who have medical problems; and women who are exposed to hazardous substances while they are pregnant.

Teratogens are substances or circumstances that can harm the fetus. Teratogens are usually most harmful during the first trimester, when the fetal organs form. The amount and timing of teratogenic exposure is critical in determining how the baby will be affected. Exposure to some teratogens, such as radiation, during the first two weeks after conception sometimes causes an early miscarriage, and at other times doesn't affect the pregnancy at all. (This is called an "all or none" effect.)

From the fifteenth to the sixtieth day after conception (weeks four to eleven), the effect of a toxin or teratogen will depend upon which organ system is developing at the time. For example, a woman who gets German measles during her fourth week of pregnancy has a good chance of having a baby with congenital heart defects and cataracts. The same infection during the twenty-fourth week is unlikely to cause problems. The fetal brain can be damaged at any time during pregnancy, so teratogens like alcohol should be avoided throughout pregnancy.

A woman should never have an abortion because she thinks that a drug she took or a chemical to which she was exposed must have caused irreversible fetal damage. She should always consult a fetal or genetics specialist before assuming the worst.

Alcohol

Women who are alcoholic or who are addicted to drugs give birth to more than 10 percent of the babies born in the United States. Drinking alcohol during pregnancy is the single greatest—and most preventable—cause of mental retardation in the United States. Drinking alcohol when pregnant should be avoided, as it can cause fetal alcohol syndrome (FAS) and is associated with higher rates of miscarriage and complications. Fetal alcohol syndrome occurs once in 750 births, and it involves developmental delays, learning disabilities, behavioral problems, heart defects, short stature, and a characteristic facial appearance. Even having one alcoholic drink every day while pregnant is associated with having a low-birth-weight baby. On the other hand, if a woman had a few drinks before she realized she was pregnant, and one or two during her pregnancy, it should not cause undue concern. Similarly, the small amount of alcohol in herbal tinctures that are taken by eyedropper are no cause for concern.

Breast Implants

Silicone implants have not been found to result in higher rates of birth defects. In fact, breastfeeding is safe through breasts that have silicone implants, and such milk actually has less silicone than infant formula. While some doctors feel that feeding babies through silicone-enhanced breasts may increase gastrointestinal ailments in the babies, this has not been proven.

Caffeine

Caffeine is found in coffee and tea, with black tea having considerably more than green tea. An average cup of brewed coffee has about 100 milligrams of caffeine, a cup of instant coffee about 50 milligrams of caffeine, and a cup of black tea about 40 milligrams. Caffeine is added to many soft drinks such as Coca-Cola, Pepsi-Cola, Dr Pepper, Tab, and Mountain Dew. An average cola drink has 30–45 milligrams of caffeine per serving. Ingesting more than three cups of coffee a day has been shown to increase the incidence of miscarriages.

Pregnant women should moderate their intake of caffeine, whether from coffee, tea, or caffeinated soft drinks.

Cleaners

Many home cleaning and polishing products contain petroleum distillates, benzenes, naptha, chlorinated hydrocarbons, and ammonia. All of these can be dangerous to pregnant women. It is far better (and usually cheaper) to clean with vinegar or lemon juice, or use cleaners such as chlorine-free Bon Ami and steel wool.

Exposure to chlorine products such as household bleach or swimming in chlorinated swimming pools has not been shown to harm the fetus.

Cigarette Smoking

It is best not to smoke or be exposed to second-hand smoke during pregnancy. At least four thousand chemicals are inhaled when one breathes in cigarette smoke. Many of these are carcinogenic, and they destroy vitamins B and C, folic acid, and calcium. Smoking doubles the risk of having an ectopic pregnancy, and it increases the risk of having placenta previa and heavy bleeding during the last trimester. Nicotine narrows the blood vessels, reducing the amount of oxygen that the baby gets. This, in turn, increases the risk of premature delivery, miscarriage, low birth rate, and the tearing away of the placenta from the uterine wall (placental abruption). Smoking by mothers or fathers during pregnancy has also been linked to babies having higher rates of sudden infant death syndrome (SIDS).

Electromagnetic Radiation

Well-designed studies have not shown electromagnetic fields that are generated by high-voltage power lines or home appliances such as televisions, electric stoves, washers, or dryers to be related either to complications during pregnancy or to fetal problems. Computer screens (video display terminals) produce a minimal amount of electromagnetic radiation and have not been found to cause spontaneous abortion. Some people do recommend that pregnant women sit at least an arm's length away from others' terminals. The major problems noted with VDT use are eyestrain, prolonged sitting, and repetition injuries to the arm and wrist of the woman using the computer and keyboard. These can be reduced by resting the eyes every ten minutes, getting up and stretching periodically, using screens with reduced flicker and glare, adjusting the lighting in the room, and using an adjustable keyboard.

Environmental Substances

More than five hundred thousand chemicals are commonly used in the United States, of which sixty thousand or so are used at work. Only a dozen or so are regulated to reduce the damage they cause to the reproductive system. In 1985, the House Committee on Science and Technology reported that there were 850 known neurotoxicants, any of which could cause "devastating neurological or psychiatric disorders that impair the quality of life, cripple and potentially reduce the highest intellect to a vegetative state." Almost all of these are still unregulated.

One out of every six American children now has a problem such as autism, attention deficit disorder, aggression, learning disabilities, or dyslexia. The National Academy of Sciences suggested that a combination of neurotoxicants and susceptible genes may account for about 25 percent of developmental problems.

In one study, babies whose umbilical cords had significant amounts of PCBs did worse on cognitive tests than unexposed babies did.

Substances known as organic solvents (aldehydes, ketones, esters, glycol esters) are widely used in paints, preservatives, glues, and nail polish. They can be absorbed through the skin as well as inhaled, and most of them cross the placenta and appear in breast milk. Women who work long hours in laboratories, in nail salons, and who paint have a higher than normal risk of spontaneous abortion. Some of these substances may harm the kidneys and cause toxemia and high blood pressure in pregnant women.

Pregnancy is not the time to paint the house or the baby's nursery or refinish, varnish, or shellac the floors or furniture. Women artists should avoid painting, especially in poorly ventilated areas. If pregnant women must have their homes or floors painted or refinished, they should have others do it while they are out of the house. It is best to use odor-free, nontoxic paints. If latex is used, make sure to ventilate the area well.

Food Additives

Pregnancy is a time when many women try to eat as healthful a diet as possible. Hopefully, they continue doing so, and feed their families healthful foods, after they have their babies. For those who are interested in the long-term effects of foods, today's foods contain between ten thousand and one hundred thousand food additives! Some additives that are used in many foods, such as certified food colorings and sodium nitrite, are known to cause cancer in laboratory animals. It is best to avoid foods with chemical additives when possible.

Aspartame (Nutrasweet), saccharin, and other artificial sweeteners are not known to cause maternal illness or fetal disorders. Aspartame has been approved by the FDA for use during pregnancy and breast-feeding. Saccharin was found to cause cancer in laboratory animals when given in huge doses, but the FDA just took it off of their list of carcinogenic substances because it was not found to cause cancer in humans after all.

The artificial preservatives BHA (butylated hydroxyanisale) and

BHT (butylated hydroxytolvene) have not been seen to cause maternal or fetal problems during pregnancy.

Hair Care Products

Well over 50 percent of adult Americans dye their hair. Hair dyes painted on pregnant rats did not show any damage to their fetuses even when used in doses one hundred times that normally used by humans. Nevertheless, it is not recommended that women dye their hair during the first trimester. Some hair dyes contain heavy metals such as lead and bismuth, which can be absorbed through the scalp. These should be avoided during the first trimester. It is probably less of a problem to highlight the hair using foil because such dye doesn't touch the scalp at all.

Hair straighteners contain sodium hydroxide, which can cause permanent eye damage if accidentally splashed. Pregnant women should check the labels of hair products and avoid those that contain sodium hydrochloride. Pregnant women who want to straighten their hair should try hot-pressing or blow-drying it.

Hair permanents use ammonium and hydrogen peroxide solutions and should be avoided during the first trimester. Shampoos and vegetable dyes such as henna are considered safe for pregnant women to use. Aerosol hair sprays should be avoided.

Lead

Lead and industrial solvents have been linked to birth defects and brain damage, as well as to physical and mental developmental delays. There is no known safe level of lead one can ingest, and the more the mother ingests, the greater the risk of birth defects to the baby.

Lead can be ingested when it gets into the water in homes or apartments with old pipes, or when old buildings with leaded paint are remodeled or painted. If you live in an old building, you can find out how much lead your water has by calling your local water authority. Drink bottled water or use a water filter if necessary. If you want to paint or remodel your home, do it before getting pregnant, or live elsewhere while work is being done. If you stay in your home, you may want to have your blood tested for lead periodically.

Unfortunately, some fish now have high lead levels as well. Predator and fatty fish such as tuna, shark, swordfish, whitefish, mackerel, and bluefish often have high levels of lead, mercury, and/or PCBs. Several states have advised pregnant women not to eat more than seven ounces of tuna each week (about one average-size can) because it may contain lead. The Environmental Protection Agency has a website (www.epa. gov) that lists all state warnings about contaminated fish.

Medications

The overwhelming majority of pregnant women take at least one nonprescription drug, usually before their pregnancy is even confirmed. A recent survey of fifteen thousand women in twenty-two countries found that 86 percent of them took an average of three different drugs while pregnant. A good rule of thumb is that it is best not to take any medications during pregnancy unless they are considered to be safe and necessary. For example, there is no compelling reason to medicate a runny nose, while there may be more justification to take Sudafed for painful sinus congestion that prevents sleep. When in doubt, consult your health care practitioner about your symptoms and the medication you intend to take. She may know of a safer alternative.

ACNE

Taking retinoic acid (Accutane, Retin-A) during the first trimester is known to cause birth defects and miscarriage. It is best to discontinue using it a month or two before attempting to conceive.

ALLERGIES AND COLDS

The following are generally considered to be safe for pregnant women to take: allergy and cold medications, such as chlorpheniramine and diphenhydramine, which are antihistamines; decongestants such as pseudoephedrine and Claritin have no known dangerous effects during pregnancy. Expectorants (guaifenesin) and cough suppressants (dextromethorphan) are considered safe for short-term use in therapeutic doses. Nasal saline drops are fine. Allergy shots can be continued if necessary, but women should let the doctor know they are pregnant.

ASTHMA

Most asthma medications should be continued during pregnancy under the guidance of a doctor. Doctors generally believe that it is better for women with asthma to use medications and breathe well than not to use them and have the baby suffer from a lack of oxygen. The amount of theophylline (Theo-Dur, Slo-Phyllin, and aminophylline) in the mother's blood should be watched carefully since high blood concentrations can make the baby's heart beat too fast. Neither prednisone nor beta-agonists such as albuterol (Ventolin and Proventil) have been shown to cause birth defects.

It is not clear if the low-birth-weight babies that have been born to mothers who took prednisone resulted from the mother's condition or the drug. As with any maternal medical condition, the benefits of using any medication should be weighed against the potential for harming the fetus.

BACTERIAL INFECTIONS

The antibiotics penicillin, erythromycin, and cephalosporins (such as Keflex) are generally safe to use during pregnancy. Macrodantin (Macrobid) and fosfomycin (Monurol) may also be used, if necessary.

Sulfa drugs such as Septra and Bactrim should be avoided late in pregnancy because they can cause jaundice in newborns. Tetracycline should be avoided because it may interfere with formation of the baby's skeleton and cause discoloration of baby teeth. Streptomycin and similar medications can cause fetal hearing loss and are used only when absolutely necessary. It is best to avoid floroquinolones such as ciprofloxacin (Cipro) because they can cause problems with the baby's cartilage. Isoniazid may be used for tuberculosis.

BIRTH CONTROL PILLS

Some women take birth control pills or medroxyprogesterone (Provera) before realizing that they are pregnant. It was once feared that these medications caused fetal heart defects, but that has not been borne out. Women should not worry unduly if they took birth control pills or Provera in early pregnancy.

CONSTIPATION

Many pregnant women find themselves constipated, and the problem often worsens as the pregnancy progresses. Eating a high-fiber diet, drinking eight to ten glasses of water a day, and avoiding refined foods such as white flour, white rice, and sugar are the best ways of preventing constipation. When additional help is needed, stool softeners such as docusate calcium or docusate sodium and bulk-forming agents such as psyllium may be used. When pregnant women become obstipated ("bound up"), a glycerin suppository or Fleet's enema may be used. If these fail, manual disimpaction in an emergency room may be necessary.

Cathartics containing sodium and stimulant laxatives should be avoided as they may cause the woman to lose too much fluid and important chemicals called electrolytes.

HEADACHES

Excedrin and Anacin should be avoided during pregnancy. Tylenol is generally okay for use when necessary.

If you have migraine headaches, the newer "miracle" drugs like Imitrex and Zomig cannot be taken during pregnancy, and using anti-inflammatory drugs like Motrin is discouraged. If extra-strength Tylenol and a nap in a dark room with a cool washcloth on the forehead don't bring relief, other options may work.

Nonmedical techniques such as biofeedback, relaxation techniques, and stress management, usually taught by a psychologist, may reduce or eliminate headaches. Massage therapy is also effective for some.

Eliminating foods such as red wine, aged cheese, hot pepper, and so on may take away that which triggers attacks in some people. Consulting a licensed nutritionist may help identify food triggers so that they can be eliminated from one's diet.

HEARTBURN

Most nonprescription, sodium-free heartburn medications can be used during pregnancy. These include calcium carbonate (Tums), magnesium hydroxide, aluminum hydroxide, and alginic products. When over-the-counter antacids are ineffective, Zantac may be used judiciously.

HERPES

When herpes outbreaks during pregnancy need to be treated, acyclovir (Zovirax or Famvir) may be used. Women with recurrent outbreaks may consider taking it in their ninth month to prevent an undesirable outbreak when they deliver.

HIGH BLOOD PRESSURE

Women who are pregnant in their late thirties and forties may already have high blood pressure (hypertension) before they get pregnant. Obstetricians traditionally favor using methyldopa (Aldomet) to treat hypertension, since it has not been found to have any bad effects on pregnancy.

Angiotensin-converting enzyme (ACE) inhibitors can cause birth defects and even cause fetal death if they are used after the first trimester. Diuretics generally should be avoided. Beta-blockers (such as inderal) should be used only when necessary because they may cause a small percentage of babies to be born smaller than usual.

NAUSEA

Antinausea (antiemetic) medications should only be used when nausea and vomiting are so severe that they cause dehydration and significant weight loss. Reglan is considered to be the drug of choice; Zofran is also prescribed for vomiting that cannot otherwise be stopped. Compazine has been used for years, but few studies have evaluated its safety.

Benedictin was once taken by many pregnant women to alleviate their nausea. The company that made it eventually stopped because it was spending enormous sums of money defending itself against allegations that the drug caused birth defects. Since that time, Benedictin has not been shown to cause birth defects, and a Canadian firm is trying to reintroduce a form of the drug specifically for use by pregnant women. In the meantime, women can make their own Benedictin by taking 50 milligrams of vitamin B_6 and half a Unisom in the morning, and 100 milligrams of vitamin B_6 with half a Unisom in the evening.

PAIN

When pain medication is needed, acetaminophen (Tylenol) is generally considered to be safe throughout pregnancy when used in therapeutic doses. Aspirin and nonsteroidal anti-inflammatory drugs (NSAIDs) such as ibuprophen (Motrin), naproxen (Naprosyn and Anaprox), and indomethacin (Indocin) should be avoided, especially during the last three months of pregnancy.

NSAIDs may interfere with labor, cause a decrease in amniotic fluid, and cause fetal blood vessels to close too early. Codeine may be used occasionally if needed, but large doses taken close to delivery may result in the baby getting narcotic withdrawal symptoms. When a woman has extreme pain due to conditions such as kidney stones or surgery, stronger medications such as Darvocet, Percocet, morphine, or Demerol may be used when necessary.

PSYCHIATRIC CONDITIONS

Millions of Americans take psychotropic medications, and it is not unusual for a woman to find out that she is pregnant while taking them. The new antidepressants that are believed to inhibit serotonin reuptake, such as fluvoxamine (Luvox), sertraline (Zoloft), and paroxetine (Paxil), are not believed to cause birth defects when used in therapeutic doses. Amytriptilline (Elavil) may cause birth defects and should not be used. About 1 percent of the babies born to women who take lithium have a congenital heart defect known as Ebstein's anomaly.

Taking tranquilizers such as diazepam (Valium) while pregnant should be avoided. It has been linked to cleft lip and palate in babies when mothers took it during early pregnancy.

SEIZURES

Epilepsy is an illness that causes brain functions to change temporarily. Unfortunately, most of the commonly used antiseizure drugs— phenytoin (Dilantin), valproic acid (Depakote), carbamazepine (Tegretol) and trimethadione (Tridione)—are known to cause birth defects, and taking two or more of these drugs causes additional birth defects. Pregnant women with seizure disorders are more likely to have a child with problems even if they don't take medication, and they should be carefully counseled before getting pregnant. Doctors feel that it is much better for pregnant women to take medication that will keep them seizure-free than to avoid the drugs and have seizures. This is because the lack of oxygen to the baby that occurs during a seizure can cause placental abruption and fetal death.

Dilantin can cause a set of birth defects, known as fetal hydantoin syndrome, that affect the baby's bone and facial development and may result in the baby having a small head. Dilantin can also cause the mother to lack folic acid, so such women must be especially careful to take extra folic acid before getting pregnant.

When valproic acid (Depakote) is taken during the first trimester, it causes an increase in neural tube defects. Women who take Depakote should have carefully performed ultrasounds and alpha-fetoprotein evaluations.

Phenobarbital can cause bleeding problems and barbiturate withdrawal in the newborn, folic acid deficiency in the mother, and may cause minor birth defects as well. Even so, many doctors consider phenobarbital the least dangerous of the commonly used antiseizure medications. By comparison, trimethadione (Tridione) can cause birth defects in the babies of as many as 60 percent of the women who take it.

When it is possible to change to a drug that is less dangerous to the fetus, the transfer should be done before conception, slowly, and under the care of a neurologist. Even when pregnant women take anticonvulsants, they can have a 90 percent chance overall of delivering a healthy baby.

VAGINAL INFECTIONS

Many pregnant women get yeast infections. The best-known way to avoid yeast infections is by limiting or avoiding sugar in the diet, by eating foods or supplements with acidophilus, and by wearing panties with cotton crotches. When a yeast infection develops anyway, miconozole (Monistat 3) is an over-the-counter medication that may be used safely during the second and third trimesters (although it is probably best to insert it a little less deeply than normal). Terconazole (Terazol) and fluconazole (Diflucam) should be avoided, if possible. Terazol is absorbed from the vagina into the bloodstream. Lotrisone cream is often used topically to alleviate the external discomfort caused by a yeast infection. Douching by pregnant women is discouraged.

Two other common vaginal infections are vaginosis and trichomonas. Metronidazole (Flagyl) may be used after the first trimester, if necessary, and Metrogel vaginal cream, which is used for vaginosis, is a form of Flagyl. Clindamycin cream may also be used for vaginosis.

Microwave Ovens

Large doses of microwave radiation can damage a fetus, but microwave ovens are made with metal screens that prevent the microwaves from escaping. Moreover, microwaves can't travel long distances even if they aren't blocked if a door is defective. It is considered safe for pregnant women to use microwave ovens, provided they stand several feet away while the machine is operating.

Mercury

Mercury is most commonly ingested by eating fish. The Food and Drug Administration's guideline of one part per million of mercury in fish has been deemed by the National Academy of Sciences to be "inadequate to protect the developing fetus." A 1997 study of lakes in the northeastern United States and Canada showed that fish had far more mercury in them than had been expected. Surprisingly, the cleanest lakes had fish with the highest mercury levels. Avoid eating predator fish such as swordfish, shark, tile fish, and king mackerel. Moderate amounts of tuna may be eaten.

Nail Care

Nail care products contain alcohol, toluene, and acetone. These products are considered safe to use in moderation in a well-ventilated room, but they have been associated with higher rates of miscarriage when used by women who work in nail salons.

Pesticides

Pesticides are domestic versions of wartime nerve poisons. One of the best known, Dursban, is found in roach and ant sprays. It was just banned by the Environmental Protection Agency (EPA) in June 2000 for most household uses because it can cause brain damage, but it is still being used on fruits and vegetables. The EPA found that another popular pesticide, Diazinon, could be inhaled at well above the safe dose after exterminators spray it into cracks and crevices in people's homes. A third pesticide, chromated copper arsenic (CCA) is put on pressure-treated wood that is commonly used on desks and playground equipment. For over twenty years, EPA researchers have indicated that it is especially dangerous to pregnant women who can be exposed by breathing fumes from unfinished wood during home repair or construction. Many studies show that CCA can reduce memory and intelligence.

Ninety percent of pesticides have never been adequately tested to see if they cause nervous system damage; three-fourths have not been adequately tested to see if they cause cancer; more than half have never been tested to see if they cause birth defects; and about one-fourth have never been tested to see if they cause genetic mutations.

Some studies have shown that agricultural workers have higher rates of prematurity, toxemia, and low-birth-weight babies. Many lawn and garden chemicals are dangerous and unnecessary and should be avoided unless they are absolutely necessary. Most golf courses use pesticides, and these chemicals sometimes enter the local water supply. It is best to stay away from treated golf courses and lawns for at least twenty-four hours after they are sprayed.

Pesticide residues are also found on most foods that are conventionally grown, and in the animals that eat them. About 25 percent of the world's pesticides are used on cotton, and cottonseed oil is used in many foods that contain "vegetable oil." Many fruits and vegetables absorb pesticides through their root systems, then have waxes applied that seal in the surface sprays as well. Experts at the Environmental Protection Agency recommend eating organically raised food when possible, or peeling fruits and vegetables when conventional produce is eaten.

The malathion insect spraying that was carried out against mosquitoes carrying the West Nile virus in San Francisco in 1981 and 1982, and in New York in 1999 and 2000, did not seem to have been dangerous to fetuses.

Recreational Drugs

Smoking marijuana during pregnancy has been associated with low birth weight and premature deliveries.

Cocaine and crack should never be used by pregnant women. Using them during pregnancy increases the chances of miscarriage, premature labor and delivery, placental abruption, and birth defects. When such babies are born, they may be irritable, sleep and feed poorly, and later have learning and behavioral problems.

Taking methadone during pregnancy has not been shown to cause birth defects, but taking it near delivery can cause narcotic withdrawal in the baby.

Stress, Physical and Emotional

Women who work more than nine hours a day, or who work night shifts, have a higher than normal risk of delivering prematurely. Pregnancy and having a new baby are among the most stressful events that people undergo. Several studies have shown a strong relationship between high levels of stress and spontaneous abortion and preterm labor. The combination of a very stressful job plus working one hundred or more hours a week doubled the rate of preterm labor in medical residents (doctors-in-training). This is one reason why pregnant women should get enough rest and avoid overly long work hours.

No relationship has been found between emotional stress and birth defects, although some studies have found that women who experienced severe financial problems had a sixfold increase in low-birth-weight babies. When women who were at risk for preterm labor decreased their activity level, lightened their work schedule, and got household help, they had one-third fewer premature babies than women who did not make these changes.

Ultrasound and Noise

Diagnostic ultrasound has been in use since the 1950s and is generally considered to be safe for both mother and baby. There is no evidence that it damages the baby's hearing or any other parts of the baby.

Most studies have found no association between occupational noise and living near airports and birth defects. However, since the baby can hear in the uterus, women may want to avoid exposure to extremely loud noises such as rock bands, firearms practice, noisy construction sites, and the like.

Vitamin A

Everybody needs vitamin A or beta-carotene, which the body changes into vitamin A, in order to function. Doses of vitamin A above

8,000 (some research indicates that the threshold is above 20,000) international units are believed to increase the risk of having birth defects involving the face, skull, urinary tract, and genitals.

Beta-carotene, which is found in many fruits and vegetables, does not appear to cause birth defects. The doses of vitamin A in prenatal vitamins are safe. A daily drink of carrot or vegetable juice that contains a few carrots is also considered to be safe during pregnancy.

Retin-A (tretinoin) is a cream used for wrinkles, acne, and molluscum contagiosum. It should not be used during pregnancy, but its risk of causing birth defects is extremely low. It failed to cause birth defects when it was used on animals.

Water

Not all water is safe to drink. Many municipal water sources are known to be contaminated with pesticides, chemical solvents, and/or heavy metals such as lead, all of which are detrimental to the fetus and mother. An Environmental Protection Agency study done fifteen years ago showed that one in five Americans drank lead in drinking water that came from municipal water sources. Therefore, drinking bottled water or using a water filter can be beneficial to some women.

X Rays

Pregnant women usually know not to deliberately expose themselves to X rays. If X rays are unavoidable, what effects do they have? X rays during the first few weeks of pregnancy have an all-or-none effect, either destroying the embryo or not affecting it at all. Radiation later on in pregnancy can damage a fetus. Doctors consider ten rads to be the maximal radiation exposure that pregnant women can have, even though no major birth defects have ever been reported from radiation doses below 25 rads. Diagnostic X rays of the chest, kidney, and bones are well below that level. Pregnant women who have radiation treatment should know that the radiation can damage the fetal brain and nerves and cause stunted growth. The children that are born after exposure to significant X-radiation have higher rates of childhood cancers, especially leukemia.

While pregnant women should avoid toxins when possible, doctors believe that most chemicals and drugs are safe during pregnancy. Still, pregnant women should only take medicine when necessary.

Prenatal Screening and Diagnosis of Fetal Anomalies

*P*renatal tests that screen for fetal anomalies identify small groups of pregnant women who are more likely to have a baby with a specific birth defect. Screening tests can only give a probability or risk that a specific condition is present; they cannot give definitive answers. They are given to most pregnant women.

Prenatal diagnostic tests are procedures such as amniocentesis, chorionic villus sampling (CVS), and cordocentesis that can tell definitively if a fetus has chromosomal defects or genetic disorders. They tell 100 percent of the time if a specific baby tested will have a given disorder. Since diagnostic tests are invasive and involve a small risk of miscarriage or of hurting the baby, they are usually done only on the 5 percent of women who had positive screening tests, or on those who have a higher than average risk because of their age or other factors.

Screening usually involves finding out the mother's age and family medical history. Jewish women of Ashkenazic descent are more likely to have a child with Tay-Sachs, Canavan's disease, or Gaucher's disease. African-American women are more likely to have a baby with sickle-cell anemia, and Italian women have a greater risk of having babies with thalassemia. These women (and their husbands) can be screened to see if they are carriers of these diseases.

Although high-risk mothers generally have more than an average chance of giving birth to an affected baby, the vast majority of babies with birth defects are born to younger, apparently healthy mothers with no history of birth defects. This is because most babies born are to women under thirty-five.

Having blood tests or sonograms are safe, noninvasive ways that most women can have to see if they have a higher than usual risk of carrying a baby with specific kinds of birth defects. It is reassuring, but not an absolute guarantee that the baby will be normal. It is hard to know how accurate these tests are, but they seem to identify up to 90 percent of chromosomally abnormal fetuses.

When screening tests show that a birth defect is likely, a woman may be offered a diagnostic test such as chorionic villus sampling or amniocentesis to tell definitively if the fetus has a defect. Women who are over thirty-five, who are known carriers of a defective gene, or who have previously had a child with a birth defect are often offered diagnostic tests.

It is important to let a practitioner know if you don't want screening or diagnostic tests because the potential reassurance they might provide is not worth the potential anxiety they might cause. If you are unlikely to abort the baby regardless of test findings, there is probably no reason to have the test.

What are these screening and diagnostic tests, and why aren't they routinely given to all women?

First Trimester Screening (Ultrascreen)

Early screening for Down's syndrome is now available using a combination of ultrasound examination and blood tests done between the eleventh and fourteenth weeks of pregnancy. This can be reassuring for most mothers who would otherwise not have screening tests until fifteen to eighteen weeks of pregnancy, and amniocentesis until sixteen to twenty weeks.

The ultrasound examination shows a fetal heartbeat and accurately determines how old the baby is. It can also measure the amount of fluid behind the baby's neck (called nuchal translucency). Babies with Down's syndrome and congenital heart defects usually have greater than normal amounts of this fluid.

Two chemicals in the blood are also analyzed: free Beta human chorionic gonadatropin (free Beta HCG) and pregnancy-associated plasma protein A (PAPP-A). Free Beta HCG tends to be higher than normal when the baby has Down's syndrome, and PAPP-A tends to be low. The results of the ultrasound exam are combined with the blood test findings and the mother's age in order to estimate the risk of having a baby with Down's syndrome or trisomy 18. The ultrasound with blood test identifies the 5 percent of women who are at highest risk for having a baby with Down's syndrome. Ninety percent of all babies with Down's and trisomy 18 will be born to this group of mothers, although most of the pregnancies in this 5 percent group will result in healthy babies.

The downside of the ultrascreen is that it only screens for Down's syndrome and trisomy 18. A woman who wants to know if her baby has spina bifida still has her blood drawn for an alpha-fetoprotein (AFP) analysis around week fifteen.

Women with a high risk of having a baby with birth defects need to decide whether or not to have invasive diagnostic tests, and what to do if the baby is diagnosed with an abnormality. They may want to discuss their feelings with their spouse, their practitioner, a genetic counselor, their family, and their clergy. While a diagnostic test may reveal that a baby will have a birth defect, it may be difficult to know how severely the child will be affected. In such cases, it may be helpful to find out from medical and surgical experts what one might expect, then consult people from support groups who can discuss how they dealt with their children's problems.

Chorionic Villus Sampling (CVS)

Another diagnostic test that can be done as early as ten weeks in the pregnancy is chorionic villus sampling (CVS). It involves sampling the placental tissue via a needle inserted through the woman's uterine cervix. It should only be done by someone who is expert at it, as most recently trained maternal-fetal specialists are. Like amniocentesis, which is done later, it carries with it a small risk of injuring the baby or causing it to be inadvertently aborted. Most maternal-fetal medicine specialists who do CVS feel that it is as safe as amniocentesis.

Amniocentesis

Amniocentesis is a way of sampling the amniotic fluid. It may be done as early as thirteen weeks of pregnancy, but more often it is done between weeks fifteen and eighteen. It is the test most frequently recommended to pregnant women who are thirty-five years old and over. Under ultrasound guidance, the doctor inserts a hollow needle into the amniotic sac, through the woman's belly (but not through the navel, as is commonly thought). (See fig. 3.) Less than an ounce of fluid is taken out and sent to a laboratory for analysis. Because the baby sheds cells into the amniotic fluid, these can be encouraged to grow in the lab, and then be put under a microscope to see if any abnormalities are present.

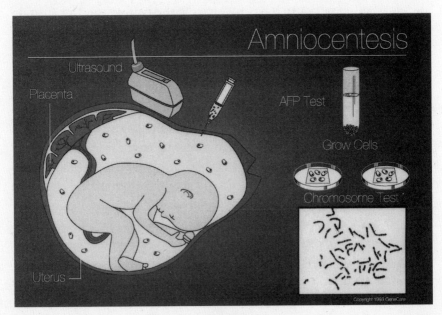

Fig. 3

Normally, it takes about two weeks for the results to be available, although newer techniques are being developed that allow for rapid read-outs.

Besides doing a routine check for certain chromosomal abnormalities, amniocentesis may also be recommended at other times. When the woman has an ultrasound between weeks eighteen and twenty, certain findings may suggest that the baby has abnormal chromosomes. These sonographic findings include swollen kidneys, a density in the bowel (known as an echogenic bowel), a specific type of cyst in the brain (choroid plexus cyst), and an umbilical cord with only two blood vessels instead of the usual three. An echogenic bowel may also show on ultrasound when the baby has cystic fibrosis or cytomegalovirus.

A choroid plexus cyst is a small, harmless, transient cyst in part of the brain. These cysts have been linked with chromosomal anomalies in 1 percent of patients, typically fetuses with trisomy 18. Such babies usually have other anomalies as well. This cyst does not suggest a higher than normal risk of a Down's baby.

When an umbilical cord lacks one blood vessel, it is recommended that a fetal echocardiogram be done to see if there is an associated heart defect. The practitioner will want to see if the baby is growing at a normal pace, and will do non-stress tests with sonograms toward the end of the pregnancy. The practitioner may recommend amniocentesis when a blood vessel is missing because there is a slightly increased chance of the baby having chromosomal abnormalities.

When the baby has swollen kidneys (hydronephrosis), serial sonograms are done to make sure that the condition does not get worse. If it does, early delivery may be warranted. In rare cases, the condition gets worse long before the due date, and fetal surgery may be necessary. Amniocentesis is usually recommended to rule out the small chance that there are concurrent chromosomal problems.

Alpha-fetoprotein

Alpha-fetoprotein (AFP) is a protein made by the fetal liver. There is a lot of AFP in the baby's blood, and a small amount crosses the amniotic membrane and passes into the mother. When the baby has an open neural tube defect, a lot of its AFP goes into the amniotic fluid, which results in an abnormally high amount of AFP in the mother's blood.

The mother's blood can be tested for AFP between fifteen and eighteen weeks of pregnancy. A small amount of blood is taken from the mother's vein and is sent to a lab for analysis. Results are usually available in about a week. This screening will identify women who have a high risk of having a baby with a neural tube defect (NTD). Most of these high-risk mothers will have healthy babies, but 98 percent of the babies who have NTDs will be born to this group of mothers.

While AFP is high in mothers of babies with neural tube defects, it tends to be lower than normal when a woman is carrying a baby with Down's syndrome or trisomy 18.

It should be noted that some AFP tests show high amounts of AFP for no known reason. Even if ultrasound and amniocentesis confirm a normal pregnancy, these babies have a higher than average risk of toxemia, preterm birth, decreased amniotic fluid, and being small for their gestational date. The high AFP should alert the practitioner to keep a closer watch on such pregnancies. Whether this reflects a defect in the placental-uterine connection is currently being researched.

Other Blood Screening Tests

There are three other blood tests that are commonly used to screen pregnancies that are at risk for Down's syndrome and trisomy 18. HCG (human chorionic gonadatropin) is a hormone made by the placenta that helps the fetus grow. When a baby has Down's syndrome, there is more HCG than usual; when trisomy 18 is present, there is less HCG than usual.

During pregnancy, the placenta makes a protein called free Beta HCG. This is the most specific biochemical marker for Down's syndrome. Free Beta HCG is high when the baby has Down's, and low when the baby has trisomy 18.

Unconjugated estriol is a hormone made by the placenta and the fetal liver. Its levels are slightly lower than normal when the baby has either Down's syndrome or trisomy 18. Even though estriol is a relatively poor indicator of Down's syndrome, many American laboratories use this along with AFP and HCG as a triple screening test for Down's syndrome.

All of the above tests can be done from blood drawn at the same time as for the AFP test. When these tests are done together, they identify the approximately 5 percent of women who are most likely to have a baby with Down's syndrome. As with neural tube defects, most of these mothers will have babies who are healthy, but 50–75 percent of all babies with Down's syndrome will be born to mothers in this group.

Neural Tube Defects

Neural tube defects (NTDs) are birth defects that affect a baby's head and spine. They occur when the neural tube—the part of the embryo that becomes the brain and spinal cord—stays open instead of closing during the first month of pregnancy. NTDs are among the most common of the serious birth defects, with one or two occurring among every one thousand live babies. The cause is unknown, and 95 percent occur in families without a history of these defects. It is known that when women take .4 to .8 milligram of folic acid before they get pregnant, and during the first few weeks of pregnancy, the incidence of spina bifida is much less. This is why any women who might get pregnant should be sure to get at least .4 milligrams of folic acid in their diet or in vitamin supplements every day. Women who already had a child with spina bifida should take .4 milligrams of folic acid before conceiving and early in pregnancy. Women who take antiseizure medications, which are known to increase the risk of having a baby with NTDs, should do the same.

Open spina bifida is another form of NTD, where some of the spine remains open. The consequences depend upon where the opening on the spine occurs. In general, when the opening is very low on the spine, the problems may be relatively minor. When the opening is higher on the spine, the problems can be very serious. They include paralysis, lack of bowel or bladder control, and in some cases, mental retardation or even death.

Fetal Umbilical Cord Sampling

One of the exciting advances during the past fifteen years has been the development of a relatively safe technique that allows fetal blood to be sampled. It is called cordocentesis, or percutaneous umbilical cord sampling (PUBS). It is a way of doing a blood test on a fetus as early as eighteen to twenty weeks, just as blood tests are done on adults.

It is done in a way that is somewhat similar to amniocentesis. The mother lies on her back on an examining table. Her belly is then swabbed with Betadine solution to make sure that the procedure is done under sterile conditions. A skilled fetal specialist, referred by her health care practitioner, will use continual ultrasound to guide the insertion of a thin needle through the mother's abdomen into the baby's umbilical cord near the place that it exits the placenta. A small amount of fetal blood is taken from the cord, and the needle is withdrawn.

The most common reason to do a cordocentesis is to quickly test the baby's chromosomes. Other reasons to do it are:

1. To treat fetal anemia. When an Rh-negative mother had a prior Rh-incompatible pregnancy, and did not get a Rhogam shot, she can develop antibodies to the next Rh-positive baby she carries. That would destroy the baby's red blood cells, causing fetal anemia. This problem gets worse with each successive pregnancy. Transfusing a fetus with Rh disease is the most common treatment done using cordocentesis.

2. To make sure the baby does not have a fetal infection such as cytomegalovirus (CMV) or toxoplasmosis. (See chapter 15.)

3. To count platelets. Platelets are parts of the blood that help it clot. Blood is actually a liquid with three parts: red and white blood cells and platelets. Red cells carry oxygen, white cells fight infection, and platelets make blood clot when necessary, such as when there is a wound.

A low platelet count could result in torrential bleeding called hemorrhage. When a mother has a low platelet count, it needs to be determined if it is because she is pregnant or because she is making antibodies against her platelets. If she makes antibodies against her platelets, some may cross the placenta and attack the baby's platelets. If cordocentesis determines that the baby's platelets are dangerously low, a cesarean section will be planned to make sure that the trauma of birth doesn't cause the baby's brain to bleed.

4. To give medication to the fetus. When a fetus has an irregular heartbeat, vital medication can be injected into his bloodstream using cordocentesis.

While most chromosomal anomalies and many other fetal problems can now be diagnosed, all of the tests in the world cannot guarantee a "normal" child. Some babies with normal chromosomes and alpha-fetoprotein levels develop into children with serious physical and/or developmental problems, such as autism and pervasive personality disorders.

CHAPTER FOURTEEN

Medical Problems during Pregnancy

Accidents and Injuries

Pregnant women, like anyone else, can be in car accidents or get injured in other ways. When trauma to the abdomen occurs, placental abruption poses the biggest danger. The separation of the placenta from the uterine wall causes massive bleeding. Preterm labor and fetal distress without placental abruption can also occur.

One way of protecting the abdomen from trauma is to wear seat belts when traveling by car. The lap portion should be secured under the belly, while the shoulder part is fastened above it.

Pregnant women frequently fall or get hit on the abdomen, and small children kick or throw toys at them. They then worry that these events could harm their baby. It is almost impossible for a baby to be hurt during the first trimester because it is well protected behind the bony pelvis that shields it.

A woman who has an abdominal injury after twenty-four weeks of pregnancy, such as in a car accident, should have a fetal heart monitor for at least four hours if the uterus isn't contracting, and as many as twelve hours if it is. Ultrasound is used to see if the fetus is doing well.

143

Most abruptions will take place within the first four to six hours after an accident.

Unfortunately, women who have been victims of prior spouse abuse are likely to be beaten again when they are pregnant. Any woman who is hit by her husband should tell her caretaker, and contact a hotline or support group for domestic violence.

Pregnant women who are fire victims need to be concerned with two things: how much of the body was burned, and whether they inhaled smoke. Smoke delivers carbon monoxide to the fetus, so mothers who inhaled smoke should get oxygen as soon as possible.

Insect stings by yellow jackets, wasps, or hornets cause pain, itching, and swelling. Stingers that are left in the skin should be removed, and ice can be applied. Antihistamines will reduce the symptoms.

A woman who was stung many times may get swelling all over her body and have diarrhea, vomiting, fever, flushing, and wheezing; she may even lose consciousness. Such women are usually hospitalized for a day or two, where they are given epinephrine, intravenous steroids, oxygen, and fluids as needed.

Dog bites are a problem because bacteria introduced into the victim's body may cause infection. The wound should be washed well with saline, and dead tissue should be removed. Antibiotics are normally needed only if the skin was punctured. Rabies shots may be gotten if necessary.

Allergies

Environmental allergies to substances such as pollen, dust mites, animal dander, and molds are common. Allergies may be helped by removing objects that collect dust, such as drapes and rugs, by regularly cleaning surfaces and floors, and by not keeping animals or flowers in the house. Keeping the windows closed (and using air conditioning, if necessary) when pollen counts are high, and in autumn when molds proliferate on leaves, can also help.

Food allergies and sensitivities can be helped by identifying the offending substances (often dairy products, wheat, soybeans, peanuts, citrus, nuts, or corn) and avoiding them.

Pregnant women can take over-the-counter antihistamines, including Claritin, judiciously, and may also continue taking allergy shots. They should let the allergist know if they are pregnant.

Breast Lumps

Pregnant women should continue to examine their breasts every month. This is done by first getting the skin wet and soapy in the shower or bath, then pressing hard in a circular pattern around the breast with the flat part of the second and third fingers of the opposite hand. This should be repeated after drying off, lying down with the same arm raised over the head as the breast that is being examined. Tell the health care practitioner if you find a lump, which is most likely to be benign. A mammogram will not be done (it would be almost useless anyway because breast tissue is so dense during pregnancy) but the lump may be aspirated or biopsied if necessary.

Cancer

Pregnant women are rarely diagnosed with cancer. The overwhelming majority of cancers that do occur, with the rare exceptions of malignant melanoma and sarcoma, do not spread to the fetus, and pregnancy does not seem to increase a woman's chances of having a recurrence of breast cancer or to hasten a cancer's progression.

Mastectomy is the treatment of choice for breast cancer occurring during pregnancy. It is impossible to adequately shield the fetus from the radiation treatment generally given after lumpectomy.

Some women with uterine cancers have had their cancers temporarily reversed with progesterone therapy, conceived and delivered a child, and then had their uterus removed.

Chemotherapy, such as methotrexate, has been shown to cause birth defects and miscarriage when given during the first trimester. During the second and third trimesters the effects are not known, although there is a higher incidence of small babies and those with bone marrow suppression. It is preferable to delay treatment until after delivery, whenever possible. Breastfeeding while undergoing chemotherapy should be avoided.

Carpal Tunnel Syndrome

One of the most common complaints of pregnant women is having a sensation of pins and needles, pain, or weakness in their hands. This carpal tunnel syndrome occurs when the nerve that runs down the arm to the hand gets compressed as it travels to the swollen wrist. This median nerve, as well as some tendons, pass through a tunnel in the wrist that is formed by several bones. The nerve gets squeezed by anything that crowds this already-snug area. The swelling and water retention of pregnancy cause this crowding, resulting in the uncomfortable symptoms of nerve compression.

At first, women will feel pins and needles, which may be made worse when the hand is moved. A few months later, the wrist and hands may feel quite painful, even numb. If this continues for a long time, the hand may become weak and some of its muscles may even shrink (atrophy). When the woman gives birth, the condition usually goes away.

What can be done about it during pregnancy? Initially, immobilizing the wrist with a splint helps, and massage by an expert massage therapist may also help. When there is severe pain during pregnancy, or if the condition doesn't go away after childbirth, steroids are usually injected into the carpal tunnel, bringing immediate relief. Unfortunately, more than half of the time a relapse occurs within a few months. When the above measures don't bring relief, surgery is usually done.

Cervical Conditions

If a pregnant woman has an abnormal Pap smear, the cervix is examined with a special magnifying glass (colposcopy) to see if there is inflammation or atypical tissue. A biopsy may be done, if necessary.

Most cervical cancers are diagnosed in a preinvasive state, in which case Pap smears and colposcopy are done every two to three months. If no progression to invasive cancer occurs, treatment can be delayed until after childbirth.

If invasive cervical cancer is found, the woman, her obstetrician, and an oncologist need to make a complex decision together, since the treatments of choice—radiation or surgery—can cause birth defects or kill the fetus.

Women with cervical cancer usually deliver by cesarean section to avoid the risk of hemorrhage or spreading the cancer.

Dental Conditions

It is important to take care of one's teeth and gums during pregnancy because pregnant women are more prone to having normal congestion of the gums, as well as gum inflammation (gingivitis) and bleeding. Pregnant women often find that their gums bleed when they brush them. If plaque is removed by brushing and flossing within twenty-four hours of eating, some of these problems can be prevented. If gingivitis is left untreated, it can cause gum bleeding, pocketing, and loosening of the teeth. The good news is that pregnancy does not worsen cavities.

Studies have shown that when pregnant women have periodontal disease affecting as few as two teeth, they are up to seven times more likely to deliver preterm, low-birth-weight babies. When "attachment loss" affects 30 percent or more of the mouth, the risk of preterm labor is even greater. Therefore, women should try to have their periodontal problems taken care of before they get pregnant. Research is now investigating whether periodontal treatment during pregnancy reduces the risk of preterm labor.

It is important for pregnant women to have regular checkups and dental cleanings every six months without routine X rays. Infrequent cleanings and tartar buildup cause inflammation that can lead to gingivitis. If X rays are necessary to diagnose or treat a problem, they may be done with a lead shield on the woman's abdomen. The dose of radiation used in dental X rays is a fraction of the amount needed to cause birth defects. Using a lead shield means that the amount of fetal radiation exposure is minuscule.

If a woman needs antibiotics before having dental procedures, she may take penicillins, cephalosporins, and erythromycin. Tetracycline should never be used during pregnancy as it can cause staining of fetal teeth. When an anesthetic is needed before having cavities filled or when a root canal is done, lidocaine or novocaine may be used. Some practitioners advise not using epinephrine but there is really no contraindication to its limited use.

Nitrous oxide may be used for dental procedures in a concentration of less than 70 percent.

When dental procedures such as extractions cause lingering pain, extra-strength Tylenol should be used. If that isn't effective, Percocet, Darvocet, or codeine may be used as well.

A good rule of thumb is that pregnant women should take care of all dental problems that require attention, but they should not have any unnecessary cosmetic procedures such as teeth whitening or bonding. Bridges and crowns are also best delayed until after pregnancy. If a problem needs to be addressed, there is probably a way to do it safely during pregnancy. Nonetheless, lying back in a dental chair is not advised during late pregnancy because the pregnant uterus presses on the main blood vessels, which will reduce blood flow to the body.

Diabetes

Diabetes is a condition in which the pancreas doesn't make enough insulin or the body can't effectively use the insulin that is made. Insulin is a hormone that enables glucose, a form of sugar, to get into the body's cells so that it can be used for energy. In diabetics, sugar builds up in the blood until the kidneys can't filter it all out. This causes some diabetics to urinate frequently and be extremely thirsty.

There are two types of diabetes: Type I occurs in childhood, and such diabetics require insulin throughout their lives. About two in one thousand women have this type of diabetes before getting pregnant. Type 2 is not insulin-dependent. It occurs in adulthood, and affects about two in one hundred women before they become pregnant.

Gestational diabetes develops in about 3–5 percent of women when they are pregnant. They do not have preexisting diabetes, and it usually goes away after the pregnancy ends. However, women who need to take insulin do have a higher chance of remaining diabetic, or of developing it after the baby is delivered. It sometimes occurs in otherwise healthy women because the placenta makes hormones (human placental lactogen and progesterone) that cause the condition. These hormones oppose the effects of insulin. Until the placenta gets large enough to make a lot of hormone (around twenty-four weeks of pregnancy), gestational diabetes is not usually a problem. From that point on, gestational diabetes can potentially cause fetal problems.

Women normally take a glucose challenge test between the twenty-fourth and twenty-eighth weeks of pregnancy. Women with a high risk of having diabetes, such as those who previously had gestational diabetes or those who previously gave birth to a baby weighing nine pounds or more, should also take a glucose challenge test earlier in pregnancy. This screening test identifies women who might have gestational diabetes. It is done by giving a woman a sugary drink with 50 grams of glucose in it, after which she relaxes for an hour. Blood is then drawn from her arm, and the amount of glucose in it is measured. If it is more than 135 mg per 100 milliliters, she takes a three-hour version of the same test, called a glucose tolerance test. It is more definitive than the screening test and, if abnormal, it shows that the woman has gestational diabetes. She is then told how best to keep her blood sugar normal by eating an appropriate diet and by taking insulin, if necessary.

Sometimes, gestational diabetes can be managed by proper diet alone. This requires keeping the woman's fasting sugars normal (under 95 mg. per 100 milliliters), and regular sugar levels under 120 milligrams per 100 milliliters. If that is done, the baby has only a slightly increased chance of having complications. If gestational diabetes is poorly controlled, the baby may become very large (fetal macrosomia). It becomes fat, with an abdomen and shoulders that are disproportionately large as compared to the head. This can lead to shoulder dystocia, difficulty delivering the baby's body once the head has exited the birth canal.

Newborns of diabetic mothers need to be watched carefully after birth, as their blood sugars may plummet dangerously low. This is because their mothers' high sugar levels caused them to develop much bigger pancreases than normal in order to defend against the excess sugar in the uterus. These babies also have a higher risk of lung immaturity.

Most specialists believe that pregnant women with high fasting sugars are high risk. When fasting sugar is high, or when dieting alone doesn't keep after-meal sugar levels normal, women should get insulin and have frequent ultrasounds and non-stress tests.

Women with gestational diabetes in one pregnancy have a greater chance of getting it again subsequently. They also have a strong chance of developing diabetes later in life (especially if they are overweight). If they need to take insulin, some specialists believe that increases the risk of becoming true diabetics. Women who have had gestational diabetes, or who have delivered a very large baby suggesting the possibility of undiagnosed diabetes, are tested for diabetes in the first trimester of the next pregnancy, and again at twenty-four weeks if the first test was normal.

Diarrhea

Diarrhea is very watery bowel movements that may be caused by viruses, bacteria, parasites, toxins, or conditions such as colitis. Diarrhea usually runs its course without posing problems to the mother or fetus. The woman simply needs to stay hydrated.

When the diarrhea is very severe or is bloody, precise diagnosis, sometimes requiring a stool culture, is necessary. If the woman recently took antibiotics, then got severe diarrhea with abdominal pain, the *Chlostridium difficile* bacterium may be producing a toxin. This bacterium proliferates when antibiotics wipe out the "good" bacteria that normally keep it in check. When that happens, the woman needs to take another antibiotic to wipe out the chlostridium. Diarrhea that is caused by bacteria such as *E. coli*, salmonella, and shigella usually stops on its own.

Diarrhea can best be avoided by practicing good hygiene, eating fresh, well-cooked food, and being careful about where and what one eats out.

Gallstones

The prototypical gallstone patient has the four "F's"—female, forty, fat, and fertile. Pregnant women have more gallstones than others. Attacks announce themselves via severe pain in the upper right abdomen, sometimes radiating to the back, often accompanied by nausea and vomiting.

Gallstones are best diagnosed by ultrasound. When women are pregnant, they are treated with intravenous fluids, painkillers, and antibiotics. They are then sent home with instructions not to eat fatty or spicy foods, and surgery is delayed until after childbirth. If the gallbladder must be removed from a pregnant woman, it should be done by a highly skilled, experienced surgeon. Medication to prevent labor should be given when a woman undergoing surgery is twenty or more weeks pregnant.

Headaches

Headaches are one of pregnant women's most common problems. Headaches are common in reproductive-age women anyway, with as many as three-quarters of migraine sufferers being female. These headaches seem to be related to hormones and the menstrual cycle.

Migraines occur on one side of the head, with pain caused by stretching of the arteries there. When migraines occur, the woman may also lose her appetite, be nauseous, or vomit. Migraines are often preceded by a telltale "aura," a state of altered consciousness that lasts up to an hour. It can include visual hallucinations, blind spots, extreme light sensitivity, and a feeling of pins and needles. A woman with new and severe migraines should consider having a neurologic evaluation to make sure that something more sinister, such as a brain tumor, is not at work.

The good news is that most pregnant migraine sufferers find their headaches occur much less often, if at all, starting around the end of their first trimester. The bad news is that Imitrex, the most popular medication used to treat migraines, cannot be used during pregnancy. Ergotamine, another good medication, cannot be used during pregnancy either, because it causes uterine contractions. Fiorinal and ibuprophen should be avoided if possible. Tylenol may be used when needed, and nonmedical treatments should be tried. Determining what foods and additives, if any, trigger migraines, and avoiding those foods, can be extremely helpful. Some common culprits are red wine, nitrites, aged cheese, caffeine, alcohol, and monosodium glutamate.

Tension headaches are the most common type of headache in pregnant women, and they don't improve during pregnancy. They typically occur on both sides of the head, where they may cause a feeling of pressure and tightness over parts or all of the head. They are not preceded by an aura.

Biofeedback and relaxation techniques, changing lifestyles, and stress management can be helpful in reducing or eliminating both migraines and tension headaches. Some psychologists are specialized in helping people use these techniques so that they can reduce or eliminate headaches.

Hemorrhoids

The constipation of pregnancy together with the uterus pressing on the pelvic veins causes varicose veins of the rectum, called hemorrhoids. They get worse during labor, then gradually get better, but never completely disappear. Surgery is only necessary if they become very painful, hard, and blue (a form of thrombosis).

Hernias

Inguinal hernias may announce themselves during pregnancy by causing groin pain that goes away when the woman changes position or stops the activity that brought on the pain. Since changes of normal pregnancy can mimic the pain and swelling caused by hernias, either condition is treated the same way. The woman should rest as much as possible. After childbirth, a surgeon can diagnose if there is a hernia, and surgery can be done if necessary.

An umbilical hernia is a defect in the navel that can be dangerous if something gets stuck there. Once the pregnant uterus reaches the navel at twenty weeks, it prevents the abdominal organs from entering the defect in the navel, and it is almost impossible for even a large umbilical hernia to cause problems. The hernia should be repaired after all postpartum healing has occurred because there is a greater risk of recurrence if repair is done at the same time as a cesarean section. The surgery can be done through the same incision if a woman has a tubal ligation.

Lice

Lice are tiny parasitic insects that attach to hair on the head, body, or pubic area. The adults eat their hosts' blood, and the saliva from their bites causes itching. Lice lay little whitish eggs that stick to clothes, bedding, and hair. Lice have become so common in children that schools and camps do routine lice checks. Pregnant women, especially teachers, can be easily exposed.

Pubic lice are usually sexually transmitted. They leave telltale signs of tiny red dots on a woman's panties.

Kwell should not be used by pregnant women. Rid and Nix may be used on pubic and body lice. Nix is a medicated cream rinse that is put on the head after shampooing, then rinsed off ten minutes later. The hair is then combed with a small, fine comb to remove nits.

After treatment, all clothes and bedding should be washed in hot water. Anything that could touch a person but can't be washed should not be used for two weeks, during which time all the lice on it will die.

Ovarian Cyst

Many ovarian cysts that are discovered during pregnancy will disappear by the end of the first trimester. The overwhelming majority of those that persist into the second trimester are benign, although between 2 and 6 percent will turn out to be malignant. Sonograms can help diagnose which are which.

If surgery is needed, it is normally delayed until after sixteen weeks. This gives the cyst time to shrink, and it ensures that the corpus luteum is not removed while its hormones are still needed to maintain the pregnancy. Also, this gives a spontaneous miscarriage time to occur, as these happen anyway during the first trimester. Waiting also avoids irritating the uterus, which is more sensitive and prone to contractions during the first trimester.

Pinworms

Pinworms are white worms that look like little white threads. They live in the intestines and emerge from the anus at night to lay eggs, sometimes causing severe rectal itching at those times. It may get into the vagina and vulva of pregnant women and cause itching there.

Some doctors think that one should defer treatment of pinworms until after pregnancy. Because of the discomfort, and the very tiny risk of a complication such as appendicitis, many treat it with a single dose of Vermox.

Rh Disease

Most people have a certain protein, called the Rh factor, on the surface of their red blood cells. These are called Rh-positive (Rh+). A person who lacks this factor will make antibodies to fight it if they are exposed to it, such as by getting the wrong type of blood during a transfusion. The body then stores the equivalent of the invader's "mug shots" so that a repeat invasion will result in a swifter, deadlier response.

If a mother and father both have Rh-negative (Rh−) blood, she will not make Rh antibodies to a fetus. If the father has Rh+ blood, though, the baby can also be Rh+, and the mother can develop antibodies to her own baby. Women do not make enough antibodies for this to be a problem during a first pregnancy because most of the exposure to the baby's blood only occurs at delivery. Then, a significant amount of the baby's blood mingles with the mother's. By that time, the baby is outside her body, and so is unaffected.

Early in the next pregnancy with an Rh+ baby, the mother may make lots of antibodies that attack the Rh protein on the fetal red blood cells, thereby destroying those cells. The resulting fetal anemia can lead to severe swelling, heart failure, and even death if it is left untreated.

This is one of the many areas of medicine where a simple preventative measure has almost completely eliminated a problem. Since the 1960s, Rh− women with Rh+ partners, who are pregnant for the first time, are given an injection of Rh protein antibodies. This Rh-immune globulin, in the drug Rhogam, prevents women from making their own antibodies that attack fetal red blood cells. Rhogam doesn't attack the fetal blood cells, either, and these antibodies die off soon. When Rhogam is given at the crucial times when the mother is exposed to significant amounts of her fetus's blood, they will prevent her from making antibodies.

The most common times for fetal blood to enter the mother's bloodstream are: when she miscarries or has an abortion; when there is an ectopic pregnancy; when there is any significant bleeding that might come from the placenta during pregnancy after the first trimester; after any invasive procedure such as amniocentesis, chorionic villi sampling (CVS), or cordocentesis; when there was fetal manipulation that might have caused bleeding, such as trying to turn a breech fetus head-down (external version); and during fetal demise, when a lot of fetal blood might enter the mother's bloodstream.

Rhogam is given to at-risk mothers at twenty-eight weeks of pregnancy, because of minute amounts of fetal blood that escape during pregnancy. The mother's blood is drawn first to see if she has not already started making antibodies to her baby's blood. If she has, giving Rhogam will not help.

Most doctors do this test when a woman gets her glucose challenge test at twenty-four to twenty-eight weeks. If the blood test shows that she has no antibodies, she gets Rhogam at her next visit.

Since it is so difficult to know if a fetus is Rh+, all babies have their blood typed at birth. If it turns out the baby was Rh− all along, the mother needs no further Rhogam. If the baby is Rh+, the mother gets a Kleihauer Betke blood test, which measures how much of the baby's blood entered the mother's so that an appropriate amount of Rhogam can be given. Rhogam must be given within seventy-two hours of birth or miscarriage or it is too late to give it.

If the mother never got Rhogam and has already started making antibodies, what can one do? Her antibody levels are measured, and when they reach a crucial level, either amniocentesis or cordocentesis is done to measure the baby's blood count. A cordocentesis can verify the baby's blood type immediately, as well as allow a transfusion to be done through the same needle if necessary. Giving the baby blood will keep him alive until a safe delivery can occur, or until his condition deteriorates and an early delivery is done.

Toxemia

One reason why prenatal care is important is to make sure that toxemia doesn't cause a catastrophe. Toxemia is a form of high blood pressure where the woman's arteries spasm and constrict all over her body in reaction to pregnancy tissue. It rarely occurs before the twentieth week of pregnancy. It causes high blood pressure, protein that spills over into the woman's urine, and significant swelling. The cause is unknown, and the only real "cure" is to deliver the baby. If that isn't done, toxemia results in seizures.

When a toxemic woman's arteries constrict, the placenta may not get enough nourishment, or it may even tear away from the uterine wall. This may cause the baby to grow poorly or necessitate preterm delivery.

Toxemia mostly occurs with first deliveries, although women with a new husband, very young teens, and those who are pregnant with multiple fetuses also have a higher than normal risk. Toxemia tends to run in families and in African-Americans, and it is more common when women have diabetes, chronic high blood pressure, and kidney problems.

A woman's blood pressure normally remains the same during the first trimester, drops slightly during the second trimester, and slowly returns to normal during the last part of pregnancy. When blood pressure rises to 140/90 or higher, it may be due to toxemia. The urine samples that the woman gives on every prenatal visit are always checked for protein. A toxemic woman will retain a lot of water, and pressing a finger into her leg will leave a lingering indentation called pitting edema. The woman will have hyperactive reflexes, such that tapping her knee will cause her leg to swing up wildly. If blood tests show that she has too few platelets and a dysfunctional liver, she must be delivered soon. Having a severe headache that doesn't get better after taking Tylenol may be a warning that a seizure will follow. Bad pain in the upper right abdomen is also an ominous sign that warns the practitioner to expedite delivery.

When blood pressure is only slightly elevated and there is minimal protein in the urine, the woman is usually told to stay in bed and lie on her side. Lying on the back will cause a heavy uterus to squeeze the biggest vein in the body (the vena cava) and interfere with blood flow to the baby. Lying on the side allows for the best blood flow, which fights the toxemia.

The baby is delivered if toxemia occurs close to the due date. Otherwise, the woman's blood pressure is watched closely. If the toxemia gets worse, she is given magnesium sulfate (the same drug that is used with preterm labor) to prevent seizures. Labor is then induced or a cesarean section is done.

Toxemic women have narrow arteries, so they don't tolerate blood loss well. That sometimes makes it preferable to do a vaginal delivery. On the other hand, severe or quickly advancing toxemia might mean that the baby should be delivered as soon as possible, in which case a vaginal delivery would take too long. Then, a cesarean section might be done.

Women with a low platelet count, including toxemic women, cannot get an epidural. The pain from a long, induced labor without anesthesia may be unendurable. So, an individual assessment of every woman's needs is made in order to determine which type of delivery will be best for her.

There are presently no medications that can prevent toxemia. It is often recommended that women at risk for toxemia rest on their side as much as possible during the day, even if they are not tired, and avoid gaining excessive weight. These precautions and regular prenatal visits are all important ways to avoid the potentially tragic effects of toxemia.

Urinary Tract Infections and Kidney Stones

Women tend to get urinary tract infections (UTIs) more than men because a woman's urethra is very short, and it is close to the vagina. Since both the vagina and the rectum have lots of bacteria in and around them, these can easily get into a woman's urethra, and from there, into her bladder. Also, since sex bumps these delicate urologic structures, bacteria in the bladder may be whipped up into a frenzy that results in an infection.

Pregnant women may be more prone than others to getting urinary tract infections. Pregnant women make more urine than usual, and progesterone relaxes the muscles of the urinary tract. The ureters, or tubes that bring urine from the kidneys to the bladder, then lose their tone and can't contract strongly. The pressure of the pregnant uterus compounds this problem, resulting in urine stagnating in the urinary tract. To add to the problem, the kidneys normally spill more sugar into the urine, which the bacteria then feast upon.

All pregnant woman feel they need to void frequently. On the other hand, women with UTIs have pain, urinate frequently, and feel the need to constantly empty their bladders even when there is little fluid there. They may also have blood in their urine. If a woman has no pain or blood in the urine, a definitive diagnosis can be made by doing a urine culture.

UTIs in pregnancy need to be treated because otherwise they may spread to the kidneys. Kidney infections are especially dangerous in pregnancy because they can make a woman very sick and cause preterm labor. When a woman with a bladder infection gets fever, chills, pain that goes into her back, and possibly nausea and vomiting, she has signs of a kidney infection and needs immediate medical help.

Drinking enough fluids, including cranberry juice, and emptying one's bladder after sexual relations are the best defenses against urinary tract infections. Nonpregnant women who are prone to UTIs are urged to take 1,000 milligrams of vitamin C a day, as this makes the urine more acidic and less hospitable to bacteria. It is not recommended that pregnant women take large doses of vitamin C. If all else fails, a few women will need to take an antibiotic every time they have sex.

*   *   *

Most medical problems that occur during pregnancy are addressed the same way they would be were the woman not pregnant. Typically, a pregnant woman will call her primary care physician when she has aches and pains or feels ill. The doctor can consult with the obstetrician if any special obstetrical concerns need to be addressed.

CHAPTER FIFTEEN

Infections and Diseases during Pregnancy

A *pregnant woman may be exposed to a variety of bacteria and viruses* that may cause illnesses and/or require treatments that could potentially affect the fetus.

Infections

GIARDIASIS

Giardia is the most common small intestinal parasite in the United States. It may cause no symptoms, or it may cause severe diarrhea and malnutrition as it injures the intestines. A pregnant woman may get it from her small children or from drinking contaminated water from outdoor sources such as streams or lakes. If a woman has diarrhea lasting for more than three days, she should be tested for *giardia*.

The initial illness lasts for up to a week. It causes gas, cramps, abdominal bloating, nausea and foul-smelling, frequent diarrhea without a fever. (*Giardia* is not usually the culprit when these symptoms occur with a high fever.) After the first week, a chronic condition develops in which the woman will feel well for a while, then have a recurrence of bad gastrointestinal symptoms.

Giardiasis doesn't hurt a fetus; resulting malnutrition affecting the woman can. Paromomycin and metronidazole are effective treatments, but should not be used until after the first trimester, if possible.

HEPATITIS B

You can get hepatitis B when the blood of an infected person gets into your bloodstream. This can happen when someone in a health field sticks an infected patient with a needle, then the same needle accidentally sticks the caretaker, thereby introducing blood from the patient into the worker. Women at risk of getting hepatitis B are nurses, doctors, dentists, and other medical workers. It can also happen when someone gets a transfusion with contaminated blood or when drug users share needles. Modern methods of screening blood have made it rare to get hepatitis from transfusions. Sexual intercourse with an infected partner can also transmit hepatitis.

Someone who gets hepatitis B can completely recover and be immune to it, or be chronically infected and be infectious to others. Rarely, in the latter case, hepatitis will cause liver failure.

The babies of women who have hepatitis B need to get immunoglobulins and a hepatitis vaccine at birth in order to keep them from getting hepatitis from their mothers.

There have been no reported risks to the fetus when the mother is given hepatitis B vaccine. Therefore, it is recommended that people get vaccinated if they work in fields where they are exposed to hepatitis B.

If you anticipate traveling to a place where medical hygiene is not optimal, consider the risks you will have of getting AIDS or hepatitis if you need a transfusion with blood that was not carefully screened, or if you get medical care in a place that has no sterile settings.

INFLUENZA

Influenza is caused by various strains of a virus and has the following symptoms: sneezing and coughing, headache, fever, general malaise, and in severe cases, difficulty breathing. The flu virus has two basic types:

Type A is a strain that changes every year, while Type B always remains the same. These vaccines contain dead viruses that are not dangerous to the fetus. Women who have chronic pulmonary disease, asthma, or poor immune systems and who are prone to getting the flu are urged to get a flu vaccine before the flu season. Doctors now recommend that all pregnant women in their second or third trimesters get vaccinated.

MALARIA

Malaria is a parasitic infection that is spread by the bite of a certain species of mosquito. It occurs in wet, warm areas where such mosquitoes breed and thrive. The primary symptoms of malaria are chills with extremely high and low fevers, sweating, and headaches.

Malaria presents a greater threat to pregnant women and their fetuses because the malarial parasite can invade the placenta.

If it is necessary to travel to countries where malaria occurs, women should take quinine daily for four weeks prior to their visit and use mosquito repellent and netting when in malarial areas. We strongly discourage pregnant women from traveling to areas where there are drug-resistant strains of malaria. Doxycycline is usually recommended in places like South Africa that have resistant strains, but pregnant women should really not take it because it can affect fetal tooth and bone growth.

STREPTOCOCCAL INFECTIONS

Group B streptococcus is related to the group A bacteria that causes strep throat. Group B streptococcus can be found in the stomach, intestines, and urinary and reproductive tracts of healthy men and women. It is usually harmless unless the person is immuno-compromised or pregnant. If a pregnant woman has a group B strep infection, her baby will probably be well protected against it until the mother's water breaks. When the amniotic sac breaks and fluid starts to leak out, the baby loses some of its protection against the bacteria, and the bacteria can make their way from the mother's vagina and rectum into the uterus. About 1 to 2 percent of babies get infected when the mother has group B strep.

A baby with an early strep infection will get sick within twenty-four hours after being born, although it could happen as late as a week after birth. These infections move quickly and the baby often dies. A late beta strep infection starts a week or more after a baby is born, and can cause blood infection, meningitis, or bone and joint inflammation. More babies survive these but the 30–50 percent who get meningitis have long-term neurological complications.

It is not clear if babies get early and late infections the same way.

Beta strep can affect a newborn suddenly, and in devastating ways, so it is important to try to prevent it. Doctors believe that high-risk patients should be screened, then treated if their test results show they have beta strep.

A beta strep culture is easy and painless to do. The caretaker swabs a cotton swab around the vagina, perineum, and rectum, then brushes the swab over a gel in a laboratory dish. The dish is kept in a lab for twenty-four to forty-eight hours, during which time beta strep will grow if the woman has it.

We recommend that all women get beta strep cultures when they are at thirty-five to thirty-seven weeks pregnant. We give antibiotics to all woman in labor if their cultures are positive. Any women who had beta strep urine infections at any time during pregnancy are also treated during labor regardless of what the thirty-six–week culture shows.

We do cultures on any high-risk women who are admitted to the hospital when their membranes rupture before thirty-seven weeks, those who have preterm labor, pregnant women with fevers, and those who already gave birth to a child with beta strep. Since getting results takes time, these women get antibiotics until their culture results are known. If beta strep is found, the antibiotics are continued. If not, the antibiotics are stopped.

Women often wonder why practitioners wait until labor to treat them for beta strep instead of doing so as soon as a culture comes back positive. First, women are treated for beta strep only to protect the baby. There is no reason to subject women to ten days of antibiotics (with all of the ensuing problems) when one or two doses during labor protect the baby. Second, giving women a small amount of intravenous medication seems to protect the fetus much more than giving ten days' worth of oral antibiotics. Third, once treated, beta strep can recur. Treating women two or three weeks before delivery gives them ample time to be recolonized by the bacteria before they give birth.

TOXOPLASMOSIS

Toxoplasmosis is a mononucleosislike illness with symptoms of general malaise, mild fever, sore throat, and headaches. It usually resolves on its own without needing any medical treatment. Since it can also be asymptomatic, women may need their blood tested to know if they have been exposed.

It is caused by a parasite called *Toxoplasma gondii*. Cats get infected by hunting infected rodents and then excrete the parasite in their feces. The parasites can stay alive for years, usually in soil. Susceptible people can get infected by eating contaminated unwashed vegetables or undercooked meat or by touching cat feces in kitty litter and the like.

Pregnant women who get toxoplasmosis may also infect their fetuses. This happens 15 percent of the time if the mother gets it during the first trimester, 30 percent of the time if she gets it during the second trimester, and 60 percent of the time if she gets it during the third trimester. However, the severity of the infection is inversely related to the baby's age. In other words, babies who get infected during the first trimester have the greatest chance of developing serious symptoms such as an underdeveloped head (microcephaly), enlarged liver and spleen, and even death. Those who get it toward the end of pregnancy are usually born without serious problems.

Toxoplasmosis is relatively rare among pregnant American women (although it is not uncommon among French women) so routine testing is not done. When a woman lives with one or more cats, we recommend testing as soon as a pregnancy is confirmed. This is done by examining the mother's immune response using blood tests that check for IgM and IgG antibodies. If she has both IgM and IgG antibodies, it shows that she was probably exposed to toxoplasmosis some time earlier and is immune to it. If she has only IgM antibodies to toxoplasmosis, there is a strong chance that she was recently infected. If the antibody test suggests a recent infection, an ultrasound can be done to see if the baby is developing normally.

Two drugs, sulfadizin and pyrimethamine, are currently used simultaneously to treat pregnant women whose blood tests show they were recently infected with toxoplasmosis. Such women take these drugs by mouth for the rest of their pregnancies.

As with many other diseases, an ounce of prevention is worth a pound of cure. Toxoplasmosis can be prevented by avoiding undercooked meat and direct contact with cat litter. If a pregnant woman must empty her cat's litter box, or work with soil, she should wear gloves if she is not already immune to the disease. Cat owners who are not immune should also try to keep their cats from roaming outdoors in places where they can hunt rodents.

Wendy was a twenty-eight-year-old flight attendant who was pregnant with her first child. When her obstetrician confirmed her pregnancy, he asked her about her medical history and her home life. Although her medical history seemed uneventful, she did own two cats. She got a toxoplasmosis blood test, which showed an elevated IgM, indicating a recent infection. It was too early in the pregnancy to use ultrasound to see if the baby was developing normally, so it was assumed that it would be best for the baby if she were treated with drugs. She ended up having a full-term pregnancy and giving birth to a baby boy. He was tested for toxoplasmosis and turned out to have it, but showed no signs of the disease. He is now fifteen months old and doing well.

TUBERCULOSIS

Tuberculosis is an illness in which one has fever, fatigue, coughing, and night sweats. It is usually contracted by inhaling bacteria in the air after an infected person coughs or sneezes. Fortunately, only a small percentage of people who are exposed will become infected. Unfortunately, a pregnant woman with tuberculosis can give it to her baby.

Tuberculosis can be screened for by injecting a small amount of tuberculosis protein into the skin and seeing if the skin is red forty-eight to seventy-two hours later. This is known as a PPD injection, and it is safe for pregnant women.

If the PPD is positive but a chest X ray shows no tuberculosis, antibiotic therapy to prevent active tuberculosis is postponed until after delivery. Active tuberculosis, identified by a chest X ray, is treated during pregnancy by giving INH, with 50 milligrams of pyridoxine to prevent neurotoxicity from the INH. Pyrazinamide, streptomycin, and kanamycin should be avoided, if possible.

Childhood Diseases

In addition to the above infections, women may get diseases that are commonly known as childhood illnesses.

CHICKEN POX

Chicken pox (varicella) is a common childhood viral disease that can be dangerous to pregnant women. If they get the disease and it spreads to their lungs, it can cause pneumonia. When a woman gets chicken pox during the first trimester, it may cause birth defects. When the disease is active around the time of delivery, the baby may become sick.

Doctors recommend that women who are not immune to chicken pox get a two-shot vaccine at least three months before getting pregnant. Pregnant women who are not immune and who are exposed to chicken pox are given immunoglobulins to help them fight off the infection. Babies are given immunoglobulins at birth if their mothers contracted chicken pox while pregnant.

CYTOMEGALOVIRUS (CMV)

Cytomegalovirus is a type of herpes infection that most people are exposed to in infancy. Young children tend to give each other CMV when they are in day-care centers or in other places where they come into close contact with one another. So many women have already been exposed to CMV by the time they reach childbearing age that 60–65 percent of them show some immunity to the disease.

Only 1–2 percent of pregnant women get infected with primary CMV. Recurrent CMV infection can also occur, but it is not usually associated with any significant problems for babies. When a mother gets a primary CMV infection, the virus will cross the placenta and enter the fetal compartment of about half the women. Only 10 percent of their fetuses will get CMV infection, of which only 9 percent of the newborns will have no symptoms of the disease.

That is the good news about CMV. The bad news is that the remaining 10 percent of babies who get CMV in utero will have serious symptoms. These include having a small head (microcephaly), accumulated fluid in the body (hydrops), developing hearing problems, mental retardation, and retarded growth.

Most mothers who get CMV infections have no symptoms. The infection is detected when IgM immunoglobulins (the type of antibody that shows a recent infection) appear in a pregnant woman's blood when it is known they were not there before. Since very few women get tested for CMV before they get pregnant, it is difficult to know when the anti-CMV antibodies were actually produced.

Laboratories still have some difficulty determining if a woman has a current CMV infection. It is not uncommon for a laboratory to say that a woman has a CMV infection when she doesn't. This is why a woman without a very good reason to be tested should not ask to be tested.

If one suspects a primary CMV infection based on a woman's known exposure, or due to specific findings on fetal sonography, the best ways of definitively diagnosing it are by doing a very detailed ultrasound and amniocentesis. An ultrasound may reveal a smaller than expected fetus with enlarged brain ventricles and with a bowel that appears as bright spots on the sonogram (echogenic bowel). Examining a small sample of amniotic fluid may also reveal a fetal CMV infection, giving a definitive diagnosis.

FIFTH DISEASE

Fifth disease is a viral illness, erythema infectious, that is usually the fifth in a series of childhood diseases. Measles is the first disease, followed by scarlet fever, rubella, Dukes', Fifth, and roseola infantum. (Dukes' is no longer considered a separate illness by most pediatricians.)

Fifth disease is caused by parvovirus B19 and it is contracted as a respiratory infection. Infected children get mild headaches, runny nose, general fatigue, and sometimes fever, followed three or four days later by a facial rash (a so-called slapped cheek appearance) that spreads to the body, arms, and legs. Once the rash appears, the child is no longer contagious. Women who are most at risk of getting Fifth disease are mothers of children who are contagious with the disease. Although schoolteachers are often exposed to Fifth disease by their students, they rarely contract it this way.

In adults, the disease usually affects the wrist and knee joints, causing arthritis. While most outbreaks of the disease occur in late winter and early spring, the B19 virus can be contracted year-round.

Fifth disease is diagnosed based on someone having the above symptoms. It can be confirmed by a blood test that shows IgM and IgG antibodies to the B19 virus in someone's blood. IgM antibodies show that a person had a recent infection, usually within the past week to ten days. IgG antibodies usually mean the person was once infected but is unlikely to have any active viruses in their body at the time of testing. If no immunoglobulins to a given disease are present, the person is probably susceptible to the disease since she has not been exposed to it yet. If both IgG and IgM antibodies are present at the same time, the person had a recent infection that may or may not be problematic for the fetus. Unfortunately, these blood tests are not always completely accurate.

Only 10 percent of the babies of pregnant women who contracted Fifth disease are at risk of having problems as a result. The problems occur when B19 parvovirus infects fetal red blood cells. This causes fetal anemia, which makes fluid build up in the baby's chest and abdomen. This is known as hydrops fetalis. If left untreated, this can cause the fetus to die.

If there is reason to think that a pregnant woman had Fifth disease, weekly ultrasounds of the fetus are done to look for early signs of problems. If the ultrasound detects fetal swelling, indicating that the baby is anemic, fetal transfusions can be done as necessary. As long as the ultrasounds don't show signs of other fetal problems, the baby has the same chance of being healthy as any other newborn.

MUMPS

Mumps is a viral disease that one can get when an infected person coughs or sneezes. Its symptoms are feeling lousy and having pain in the muscles and joints. A day or two later, the parotid glands in the throat swell. Mumps usually occurs in children, who may be treated with bed rest and cold packs on their parotid glands.

Mumps is extremely rare in pregnant women because most were vaccinated against it as children. When it occurred during the first trimester, there was a higher rate of miscarriage within two to four weeks of the time of infection. When the pregnancies continued, mumps was not linked to any problems in the fetus.

RUBELLA

Rubella, or German measles, is a disease with which many pregnant women are familiar. It is caused by a virus that one gets by breathing in droplets that someone with rubella coughs or sneezes. About a week later, a pink rash appears on the face, then spreads down the body and onto the legs and arms. The rash lasts three to five days, during which time the person might feel generally tired and out of sorts, with a fever and joint pain.

While rubella is quite mild for a child or adult, it may be devastating to a fetus, causing a small head, deafness, cataracts, cardiac defects, and mental retardation. Approximately 8–10 percent of women who might get pregnant are not immune to rubella, either because they never got the disease (which makes people immune for life) or the immunity they got from the vaccine wore off.

Since childhood rubella vaccinations may not give lifelong protection, it is recommended that every woman who might get pregnant be tested for rubella IgG. The results will show whether or not she is currently protected against rubella. If not, she should get vaccinated against rubella prior to getting pregnant. It is then recommended that she wait three months before attempting to get pregnant.

Women sometimes get vaccinated against rubella, only to find out soon after that they were pregnant when they got inoculated. The Centers for Disease Control Registry has not found rubella vaccinations to have harmed fetuses under such circumstances. To the best of our knowledge, there is very little risk to a fetus from a rubella vaccine in pregnancy, although doctors do not knowingly vaccinate pregnant women against rubella.

Tetanus

Tetanus, or lockjaw, is a disease that one can get by introducing the tetanus bacterium into parts of the body that are not exposed to air. For example, you could get tetanus if you stepped onto a dirty nail that pierced deep into your foot or if you got a deep cut on your hand from a dirty wire on a farm. The symptoms of tetanus may include muscle spasms, headache, double vision, nausea, and vomiting and they start within twenty-four hours of getting cut.

Most Americans are vaccinated against tetanus as children. The vaccine is normally given, then followed by a second dose two months later, and a third dose six to twelve months after that. Booster shots, if needed, are given every ten years after that.

If a woman thinks that she may have been exposed to tetanus, she should get a tetanus vaccine and tetanus serum as soon as possible. If a pregnant woman will be traveling to a place where modern medical care is not easily accessible, consider the fact that tetanus cannot occur unless you receive a puncture wound. If that happens, you still have eight to twelve hours to get an injection of IgG to prevent tetanus.

The three most typical situations where one should be concerned about exposure to tetanus are:

1. If you are in an accident and are thrown from a car or bicycle and get extensive cuts.

2. If you walk barefoot anywhere, including on beaches or in water, that has beer cans, metal flip tops, metal nails, and the like.

3. If you hike in farmlands or wildlife areas or visit a farm where something metal punctures you.

Few pregnant women will want to take a syringe and IgG along with them on a trip. The IgG needs to be refrigerated and must be injected if it is needed. Therefore, we recommend that a woman who is going to a place where she might get tetanus should stay current with her booster shots before she travels. There is no reason to believe that there is any danger to the fetus from either the vaccine or the serum.

Food-Borne Illnesses

HEPATITIS A

Hepatitis is a group of liver diseases that cause symptoms of nausea, vomiting, pain in the lower abdomen, general malaise, and sometimes jaundice. Hepatitis A is contracted by eating food that was contaminated when an affected person touched it after using the bathroom without properly washing their hands.

LISTERIOSIS

Late miscarriages and stillbirths are often caused by a type of food poisoning caused by the *Listeria monocytogenesis* bacterium. There are seven types of *Listeria*, two of which can cause diseases in people. While most people are naturally immune to *Listeria*, it has been linked to several serious outbreaks of food poisoning in recent years: Mexican soft cheese caused an outbreak in Los Angeles, unpasteurized cow's milk caused an outbreak in Massachusetts, and chocolate milk caused outbreaks in Wisconsin and Michigan. *Listeria* poisoning has also been caused by eating coleslaw, pork tongue in jelly, undercooked poultry, raw fish, shellfish, cold cuts, and hot dogs. The three groups of people who are most at risk for getting listeriosis are pregnant women, the elderly, and people who are immunosuppressed, such as those with HIV.

The signs and symptoms of listeriosis are not very specific. About one-third of patients have gastrointestinal problems such as nausea, vomiting, diarrhea, and lower abdominal pain. Many patients also have a fever and malaise, such as they might have with a flu. Rarely, people get complications that include meningitis, encephalitis, and brain abscesses, although meningitis is almost unheard-of as a complication in pregnant women.

Pregnant women who get listeriosis typically feel like they have a flu, with fever, malaise, and mild uterine contractions. Once the woman is infected, the *Listeria* makes a special protein called act A. This attaches itself to cells in the mother, destroys those cells, then gets into the mother's blood. It then reaches the amniotic fluid that surrounds the fetus and attacks the fetus. Fetuses have little defense against it so they die if the infection is not diagnosed and treated promptly with antibiotics. Unfortunately, listeriosis symptoms can be so subtle that most fetuses die before treatment is even begun.

Lois was twenty-five weeks pregnant when she took a coworker out to lunch. They went to a little health food restaurant where they had soft cheese, hummus, grilled vegetables, pita bread, and herbal tea. Two days later, she had contractions and went to see her doctor. The ultrasound showed a fetus with fluid in the abdomen and around her lungs, and a weak heartbeat. The doctor suspected fetal infection and did an amniocentesis. The fluid that was removed was green instead of clear, and it was cultured in a lab. Two hours later, the microbiologist determined that *Listeria monocytogenes* was in the amniotic fluid. The mother was given antibiotics immediately, and labor was induced soon afterward. Unfortunately, the baby was born stillborn as a result of listeriosis.

Alison was a thirty-seven-year-old doctor who went to a family picnic where she ate some unpasteurized cheese. That evening, she had a fever and uterine contractions. She called her obstetrician, who did an immediate amniocentesis. Half an hour later, the microbiologist determined that the amniotic fluid was loaded with *Listeria*. The mother's blood and urine were then cultured, but no *Listeria* was found there. This showed that the infection was limited to the uterus and had not spread elsewhere. The mother was started on antibiotics, then labor was induced. After the baby was treated in the neonatal intensive care unit, both mother and baby ended up healthy, although this favorable outcome is unusual.

The main sources of *Listeria* are unpasteurized soft cheeses, such as mozzarella, feta, brie, and camembert, as well as unpasteurized milk and yogurt, undercooked meat, and raw fish. Delicatessen-counter foods with mayonnaise, such as white fish salad and coleslaw, may also be risky, and there have been recent outbreaks in the United States from cold cuts and hot dogs. Since listeriosis is so dangerous to the fetus, and so difficult to diagnose, it is very important for pregnant women to stay away from potentially contaminated foods. Even though the Department of Agriculture announced in 1989 a zero tolerance for *Listeria*-contaminated foods, *Listeria* infection in pregnancy still occurs because it is hard to prevent listerial outbreaks in food.

Sexually Transmitted Diseases

HERPES

Herpes is an infection caused by the herpes simplex virus. Type 1 herpes usually affects the lips and mouth and results in "cold sores." Type 2 infection is called genital herpes and is transmitted when an infected person has sexual contact with a partner. The virus is introduced when contact is made between a herpes sore and minor cuts in the skin and mucosa of the partner's genitals, urinary opening, and/or anus. Once inside the partner's body, the virus multiplies and destroys healthy cells by forming blisters and cold sores. These sores usually appear in clusters on the genitals, buttocks, and sometimes other areas of the body. Urination may be painful or difficult. This stage of the outbreak lasts from one to three weeks, at which point some blisters open up and eventually shrink and disappear. Even though the blisters may seem to be gone, the disease is not. The remaining viruses travel along nerve roots and stay dormant indefinitely around the nerve cells.

The majority of people with herpes get recurrent infections. In severe cases, they may get outbreaks as often as every three to four weeks. Other people may be symptom-free for months or years. Recurrent infections are usually milder than the initial outbreak, and may be provoked by stress, fatigue, or concurrent diseases.

Herpes outbreaks usually start with a person feeling itching or tingling near the infected site. The blisters appear within hours. Pregnant women usually have initial and recurrent infections that last longer than other people's.

Herpes is diagnosed by a combination of clinical symptoms, blood tests, and viral cultures. Blood tests that show if the patient has developed antibodies to the herpes virus are much less reliable than collecting fluid from a blister and sending it to a virology lab for analysis.

As with other bacterial and viral infections, the fetus is well protected against herpes, and there is no danger of it getting infected until labor starts. It can get the disease once it goes through an infected birth canal. If that happens, it may get skin blisters and rarely an infected central nervous system, leading to mental retardation, paralysis, and even death.

New data show that herpes cultures on pregnant women are not useful because vaginal deliveries can be safely done even if women have documented herpes. On the other hand, cesarean sections should be done on women with herpes who have lesions in the vaginal or labial areas when they deliver. If these women have premature rupture of their membranes they should have a cesarean section as soon as possible to avoid exposing the baby to the damaging viruses.

With herpes, an ounce of prevention is worth a pound of cure. People with active herpes infections should not have sex. People can still contract or transmit herpes if they use condoms.

Acyclovir is used to control herpes by shortening the time the outbreaks last and by reducing the intensity of the symptoms. At the present time, there is no cure for herpes, although it does seem to slowly disappear as one gets older. Most people eventually stop having outbreaks altogether.

MOLLUSCUM CONTAGIOSUM

Molluscum contagiosum is an uncommon skin condition with white, firm, shiny bumps with holes in the middle. It may be sexually transmitted. Children often contract it nonsexually, while adults often get the lesions on their genital area from sexual contact. It needn't be treated during pregnancy and it poses no danger to the baby during childbirth. The lesions often go away on their own, though most people prefer to have them removed by a dermatologist.

VENEREAL WARTS

Venereal warts (condyloma acuminata) are caused by the human papilloma virus (HPV), a sexually transmitted virus. Venereal warts and HPV infections are now quite common in the United States.

Venereal warts may be only one hard, little bump, or so many that they look like little cauliflowers on the vulva, in the vagina, the perineum, and in or around the anus. Pregnancy sometimes makes the warts grow bigger and faster.

A fetus cannot get HPV during pregnancy. In very rare cases, a baby born through an infected vagina gets juvenile laryngeal papillomatosis, although a cesarean section should not be done simply to avoid this remote possibility.

Every pregnant woman's situation should be evaluated in deciding whether the warts should be treated or removed, as some warts may go away on their own after childbirth. Cutting off large warts may cause bleeding, but they can be removed with a knife or scissors, then be stitched up if necessary. At this time, there is little information about the safety of using laser surgery on warts during pregnancy.

Pregnant women may get infections and diseases, some of which may affect the fetus. Pregnant women should try to avoid circumstances through which they might contract any illnesses. If they do get ill, they should inform their primary care physician and obstetrical caretaker.

CHAPTER SIXTEEN

Gynecological Conditions and Pregnancy

There are a variety of gynecological problems that pregnant women may need to address, even though they are not caused by pregnancy.

Abnormal Pap Smear

Pregnant women get Pap smears early in pregnancy, unless one was recently done already. The woman lies on her back with her knees spread apart while the practitioner uses a metal or plastic instrument called a speculum to hold open the vagina. If the woman relaxes, there is usually only minor discomfort as some cervical cells are gently scraped off with a tiny brush and spatula. The cells are put on a slide and sent to a lab. The lab technician examines the cells to see if any look abnormal. If they do, the abnormalities rarely represent cancer cells. This is because Pap smears usually alert women to changes years before cells are cancerous, well in time to correct these changes.

Depending upon how abnormal the Pap smear is, it is either done again or the cervix is viewed through a special magnifying lens (colposcopy) in the hope that a diagnosis can be made. Biopsies are not usually done in pregnant women.

The diagnosis is rarely cervical cancer. More common is cervical dysplasia, a benign disorganization of cervical cells than can eventually lead to cancer if it is not treated. Unless a woman has AIDS, cervical dysplasia can usually wait until after delivery to be treated.

Fibroids

Fibroids are benign tumors, made up of swirls of muscle that constitute the uterine wall. They may be as small as a pea or as large as a watermelon. Fibroids become more common as women age, and they run in families. They also tend to grow due to the increased output of estrogen during pregnancy.

Most fibroids don't affect pregnancy much, although some grow so fast that they outstrip their blood supply and start to degenerate. The resulting breakdown of that tissue can cause fever, intense pain, and contractions. Treatment is bed rest, painkillers, and Indocin for preterm labor. The pain goes away within a week.

Fibroids can also stunt the fetus's growth, push the baby into a breech or transverse position, and cause preterm birth.

Fibroids shrink after childbirth. If one doesn't shrink much and it caused a lot of problems during pregnancy, a woman who wants future babies can have it removed when she's not pregnant.

Ovarian Problems

A simple ovarian cyst is a fluid-filled sac in the ovary. If one is found during pregnancy, it is usually left alone and watched because it typically goes away on its own. Sometimes, a cyst develops when the corpus luteum bleeds. The overwhelming majority of cysts that occur during pregnancy are of this kind. Ultrasounds can ascertain that they are not growing too fast and don't look suspicious, in which case surgery should be avoided.

Another ovarian problem is an endometrioma, a form of endometriosis that occurs when the ovary is lined with tissue that normally belongs in the uterus. Endometriomas don't usually grow during pregnancy.

A dermoid cyst is a benign tumor that contains fat and hair, perhaps even teeth, along with tissue that looks like it came from other organs of the body. These usually need to be removed, but almost always when a woman is not pregnant.

Malignant tumors of the ovaries are rare in pregnant women. Surgery in all of the above cases is done only when absolutely necessary. When it can't be avoided, it may be necessary to make a large cut in the abdomen so that the pregnancy will be traumatized as little as possible. The woman is watched for signs of preterm labor, and she will get medications to prevent labor before any contractions occur.

Ovarian torsion occurs when an ovary twists around its blood vessels, causing the blood flow to be cut off. Torsion is accompanied by sudden, severe pain. Rarely, an ovarian cyst can hemorrhage or rupture, spilling the contents into the abdomen. Neither of these situations is common during pregnancy.

CHAPTER SEVENTEEN

Movement and Fetal Health

*O*ne of the most exciting times in pregnancy is when the mother first feels her baby moving inside her. While fetuses move in the uterus long before the mother can feel them, babies' movements become stronger and more detectable the older and larger they become. When the movements can finally be felt they may resemble butterfly wings fluttering inside. The sensations may continue to change as the baby grows, and are perceived differently by different women.

While a baby's movements can be the most wonderful of sensations to a mother, they are also important from a medical point of view. Once the mother regularly feels fetal movements, she should alert her caretaker if they disappear entirely.

Babies' movements are not regular, and they vary from fetus to fetus. Most mothers feel their first baby move at around twenty weeks of pregnancy. Once they know what fetal movements feel like, most women can recognize these sensations by around seventeen weeks during subsequent pregnancies. By their twenty-fourth week of pregnancy, most mothers will be able to feel their babies moving every day. The main exceptions to this are when the placenta is attached to the front instead of the back of the uterine wall, in which case the placenta dampens the mother's perception of movement. Also, overweight women may have a hard time feeling fetal movements early.

Doing a Kick Count

Doctors recommend that women start a daily habit of counting fetal movements in their thirty-second week of pregnancy. They should do this once each day, preferably after eating a meal. They lie on their side and count how many times they feel the baby move during a period of ten to fifteen minutes. (Doctors call this a "kick count.") A healthy baby will usually move three to seven times during this time. As soon as a woman counts five "kicks" she needn't count again until the next day. Since fetuses may sleep for up to forty minutes at a time, a woman needn't feel anxious unless more than that amount of time passes without fetal movements.

If she cannot feel her baby move at all during a long period of time, she should contact her health care practitioner who can follow up with various tests. Kim was a healthy twenty-six-year-old mother of two normal children. Her third pregnancy was uneventful until her thirty-fourth week, when she did not feel the baby moving for about twenty-four hours. She was very worried that something had happened to the fetus. When she called the doctor, he told her to come to the office that morning.

Non-Stress Test

When she arrived, the doctor put Kim on a fetal monitor and gave her a non-stress test (NST). An NST is done by placing a belt containing an ultrasound transducer around the mother's waist for fifteen to forty minutes. During that time the apparatus measures and records the fetal heart rate, especially as it relates to the baby's movements. Just as an adult's heart beats faster during exercise or activity, so does a healthy fetus's heart beat faster when the baby exerts itself. This increase in heart rate is called an acceleration, and it is expected that a healthy fetus's heartbeat will increase fifteen beats a minute for at least fifteen seconds when the baby moves. The practitioner hopes to see at least three accelerations over a period of fifteen minutes on the NST because they show that the fetus's heart is beating normally and that the baby is reacting properly.

The absence of three accelerations doesn't necessarily mean that the baby is not healthy. For example, our heart rates are normal but they don't show accelerations when we sleep and our breathing is shallow. If the baby is asleep when its heart rate is measured, accelerations won't occur. Since fetuses may sleep up to forty minutes at a time, we don't know if the baby is fine or in trouble if the NST is done when the baby is asleep.

In Kim's case, her fetus had a normal heart rate of 150 beats per minute. (A normal heart rate of a resting adult is around 70; a fetus's heart rate is between 120 and 160 because it has to get oxygenated blood to its entire body very rapidly.) Unfortunately, her baby didn't show a single acceleration during twenty minutes of monitoring. The doctor decided to run the test for an additional twenty minutes. Still no accelerations. He then tried to wake up the baby using an acoustic stimulator.

Acoustical Stimulation

Acoustic stimulators wake up the fetus. It is well known that babies in their mothers' wombs are sensitive to the outside environment. Mothers often report that their babies in utero are more active when it is noisy outside, such as when loud music is playing or when ambulances with screaming sirens pass by. Researchers now use this information to distinguish those babies who are asleep from those who are not getting enough oxygen in the womb. The researchers place an acoustic stimulator near the part of the woman's belly above where the baby's ear should be. When the stimulator makes a loud sound, the baby usually wakes up immediately, moves, then has an acceleration. This is similar to what would happen to us when a loud alarm wakes us up.

Acoustic stimulation has been tested in a number of places and has been found to be safe if used with caution. Unfortunately, babies who are in deep sleep may still not react to it. In Kim's case, the fetal acoustic stimulator sent out three signals to her baby, but no accelerations occurred.

Oxytocin Contraction Test

The next potential option was to give the oxytocin contraction test (OCT). This involves stressing the baby a little by giving intravenous oxytocin. Oxytocin is a hormone that the woman's body makes, and it causes uterine contractions, usually for labor and delivery. Using Pitocin, the commercially prepared form of oxytocin, is not a good idea unless the fetus is developed enough to live outside the womb because the contractions can result in labor. That rarely happens because the oxytocin that causes the contractions can be stopped at any time, but it does happen about once in five thousand uses. (OCT can also be done by having the woman stimulate her nipples, which also causes her body to release oxytocin.)

When a baby has enough oxygen, its heart rate will stay stable in response to the stress of the contractions. A baby who is not getting enough oxygen will have a decreased heart rate, usually soon after each of the mother's contractions. This is similar to how an adult cardiac stress test is used. While the person exercises, the doctor sees if the heart responds normally to the stress.

Kim's pregnancy was not far enough along to risk her going into labor, so her doctor decided to try the next option—the fetal biophysical profile.

Fetal Biophysical Profile

A fetal biophysical profile takes an ultrasonic look at the baby while almost simultaneously assessing its heart rate. The doctor observes the fetus's arms, legs, and body on the sonogram to see if they are moving. Next, she assesses fetal tone by observing if the baby is stretching inside the uterus, opening or closing its hands, or making a fist. Next, she observes if the baby is exercising the muscles that it will use to breathe after it is born. This is done either by noting if the baby's chest moves up and down during a "breathing" cycle or, preferably, by looking at the fetus's belly. When babies and fetuses breathe, their bellies go in and out instead of their chests rising and falling, as happens with adults. When a fetus has breathing movements, it is a clear sign of good health.

The problem with this test is that fetuses breathe in cycles. They might breathe for five to ten minutes, then pause for forty minutes. As you might imagine, it can be a little tricky trying to catch a baby breathing and not resting.

On the other hand, this test gives much more information about the baby and its surroundings than the OCT does, and it results in far fewer times that a healthy baby is deemed in trouble. That is why the biophysical profile has largely replaced the OCT in most hospitals.

In Kim's case, the doctor applied the ultrasound transducer and waited. After ten minutes, the baby's breathing movements were finally apparent. Everyone sighed with relief.

Amniotic Fluid Index

Besides noting if the fetus shows breathing movements, bodily movements, and good tone, the biophysical profile measures the amount of amniotic fluid in the uterus. The amniotic fluid index (AFI) is computed by measuring the pockets of amniotic fluid in the lower left, upper left, lower right, and upper right parts of the uterus, then adding them together. A normal AFI is five to twenty centimeters. Less than five is too little fluid (oligohydramnios) and more than twenty is too much (polyhydramnios).

The amount of amniotic fluid is a very important factor in deciding whether or not a pregnancy is healthy. When there is too little fluid, something needs to be done—either delivering the baby or carefully monitoring the situation with observation and repeat testing.

Too little fluid is dangerous to the baby because the umbilical cord floats in it, and the cord contains three major blood vessels that get the baby nutrients and oxygen. These blood vessels get squeezed when they aren't well cushioned, and that may prevent the baby from getting enough oxygen. Also, too little amniotic fluid shows that the placenta is not doing its job (placental insufficiency). It endangers the baby by depriving it of necessary oxygen and nutrients.

A fetal biophysical score is computed after breathing and bodily movements, tone, and AFI are taken. A score of 2 is given for each measure that is normal, and a score of 0 is given for each measure that is abnormal. If there is a normal amount of amniotic fluid, if breathing movements are seen, if there are fetal muscle tone and bodily movements, a total score of 8 is given. If the NST showed three accelerations in fifteen minutes, an additional two points are given.

A baby who is in perfect health gets a score of 10. A biophysical score less than 5 is worrisome. A good biophysical score can be reassuring for a while. When it is done on the baby's due date, the practitioner may be comfortable letting the pregnancy continue for another week. When the pregnancy is already one week overdue, the biophysical profile will be done twice a week.

In Kim's case, it was apparent that the lack of observed fetal movements was due to the baby's sleep cycle, and she had no reason for concern. The doctor told her to continue monitoring the baby using the kick count. She left the doctor's office feeling reassured about her baby's health and ultimately delivered a healthy baby boy.

The ability to diagnose fetal health throughout pregnancy is one of the greatest advances of modern obstetrics and can provide great reassurance for most pregnant women that their baby is thriving.

CHAPTER EIGHTEEN

Bleeding during Pregnancy

*F*ew *things are as frightening to a pregnant woman as vaginal bleeding.* Pregnancy, after all, is the antithesis of menstruation, and uterine bleeding during pregnancy seems ominous.

Bleeding commonly occurs at any time during pregnancy and is not necessarily a cause for alarm. While any bleeding should be mentioned to your practitioner, some types of bleeding are less likely than others to be problematic.

Early First-Trimester Bleeding

It is common for newly pregnant women to have a short, light, and painless "flow" around the time that they expect their period. This "implantation bleeding" is caused by the pregnancy tissue burrowing into the thick uterine lining, causing some blood vessels to break down. The blood that this stirs up can stay inside the uterus for a while, then seep out as a light brown fluid as much as three weeks later. Unfortunately, it may not be possible to know at this time that this bleeding is not due to an early miscarriage. The embryo is so small that it can't be seen on a sonogram for another two or three weeks. That seems an interminably long wait for an anxious, newly expectant woman to know if all is truly well.

Many practitioners draw blood at this point in order to know if the mother's hormone levels are normal. If there is a good amount of progesterone and HCG, the pregnancy may be off to a good start, while a negligible amount of HCG is a sign of miscarriage. In actuality, though, many results are more confusing than helpful because in some healthy pregnancies HCG doesn't increase as vigorously as it should, while it does so robustly in some nonviable pregnancies.

The most useful reason for measuring HCG hormones early in pregnancy is to know if a suspected ectopic pregnancy is growing. If there is a certain level of hormone, the embryo must be a certain size. If it's not seen on a sonogram of the inside of the uterus, it's looked for elsewhere.

By the time a pregnancy has reached six or seven weeks after the first day of the woman's last menstrual period, vaginal bleeding may still be innocent; it may suggest an impending miscarriage; or it might be the first indication that there is a potentially life-threatening ectopic pregnancy. An ultrasound at this point can show a healthy little embryo, with a tiny heart that is beating away. If that occurs, the risk of a miscarriage plummets to only 5 percent. The ultrasound could also show no heartbeat, a too-small embryo, or no embryo at all. These all indicate that a miscarriage might be in the works.

Whenever women have very heavy first-trimester bleeding, with clots and cramping, it is almost always a sign of a miscarriage. The main exception is when a woman carries twins, and one miscarries while the other healthy one continues to grow.

It can happen that there is no embryo, yet the woman will have signs of pregnancy. This occurs when the rest of the conceptus (the placental tissue and pregnancy sac) remains and keeps up the state of apparent pregnancy. When the pregnancy is well established, more than one ultrasound may be needed to ascertain that there is no embryo because the embryo might have been so small that it was missed on the first test. The diagnosis is usually made only after a second ultrasound is done a week later and still shows no embryo, unless one knows the exact date that conception occurred, or if the pregnancy sac is so large that a fetus should be visible.

When an embryo on an early ultrasound is smaller than it should be for its age, there are two possibilities: the fetus is sick or abnormal, and will probably miscarry, or the embryo is younger than was thought. An ultrasound done a week or two later usually clarifies matters. If the follow-up shows a vigorous embryo that is appropriately bigger, it is assumed that the initial date of conception was incorrect. If there is no embryo in the uterus, and the hormone levels are those of a fetus six weeks or older, it is assumed that an ectopic pregnancy occurred until proven otherwise. (Ectopic pregnancy and miscarriage are discussed further in chapter 19.)

Late First-Trimester Bleeding

When light bleeding occurs later in the first trimester, it is often nothing to worry about, as it is left over from earlier implantation bleeding. (Still, the health of the pregnancy should be checked.) On the other hand, heavier or fresh bleeding may come from a small separation of the placenta from the uterus. If so, an ultrasound might show a blood clot sitting inside the uterus. This is called a subchorionic hematoma. It often goes away on its own, but the woman is usually advised to rest a few weeks until the blood clot gets much smaller and no longer poses a threat to the pregnancy. At least one follow-up sonogram is usually recommended to determine that the woman is "out of the woods."

Bleeding late in the first trimester may also be due to the death of a fetus. If so, this is immediately evident by the lack of a fetal heartbeat on ultrasound.

Bleeding at any time in pregnancy can come from other sources, too. For example, intercourse can cause light bleeding when the husband's penis rubs against the pregnancy-softened cervix. Also, a woman may bleed from a polyp (a small, harmless, teardrop-shaped growth) on her cervix.

Sometimes "vaginal bleeding" actually turns out to be blood from the urethra caused by a urinary tract infection, or blood from the anus caused by bleeding hemorrhoids. It is important to determine the source of the blood. If the woman noticed the bleeding while in the bathroom, she can gently explore her vagina with a tissue or tampon. If the tissue or tampon comes out clean, the bleeding is most likely from another body opening.

Second- and Third-Trimester Bleeding

Second- and third-trimester bleeding are lumped together because the reasons for vaginal bleeding usually don't change with time after the first trimester. Bleeding during the second and third trimesters often signals a problem that requires evaluation and possible intervention. Exceptions to this include the just-mentioned benign reasons for bleeding, as well as pink staining from a severe vaginal yeast infection.

Another form of benign bleeding occurs during the ninth month when there is a light bloody and mucousy discharge called "bloody show." This is due to the "ripening" of the cervix. As the cervix opens up, thins out, and softens, some blood vessels may break. Enzymes are then released in the cervix, which breaks down some of its supporting tissue. At the same time, the mucus plug in the cervix that helped protect the uterus from bacteria drops out through the vagina. As it does, it may mix with a small amount of blood that is released from the cervix. This makes the bloody "glop" of mucus that may appear at the end of pregnancy.

Some causes of second- or third-trimester bleeding are more worrisome, so any woman who has it should inform her caretaker. Some of these causes may include:

Placenta Previa

Normally, the placenta attaches to the uterine wall well above the cervix. In a condition called placenta previa, the placenta covers the inside of the cervix (see fig. 4). The problem with placenta previa is that the cervix moves and is very fibrous. This prevents the placenta from implanting as well as it does on the thicker, richer tissue of the upper uterus. When the placenta stays there until delivery, the opening of the

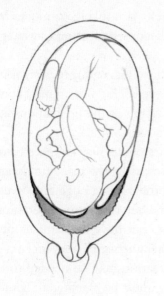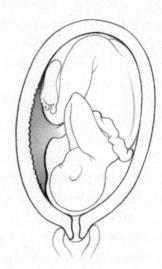

Fig. 4

cervix during labor rips into the placenta and causes life-threatening hemorrhage. Fortunately, use of ultrasound with pregnant women makes this catastrophic event extremely rare because labor is avoided when a placenta previa is known.

Placenta previa occurs in only about 1 percent of all pregnancies. It is more common among women who have given birth to a number of children, who had abortions, miscarriages, uterine curettage, or prior cesarean sections. When placenta previa stays that way at term, a cesarean section is done in order to avoid massive bleeding.

Women with placenta previa do not usually bleed until the end of the second trimester or later. When a woman bleeds during her second or third trimesters, ultrasound can determine if placenta previa is the culprit.

When placenta previa is diagnosed, it will not necessarily block the cervix for the duration of a pregnancy. As the pregnancy advances and the uterus grows, the relative position of the placenta may change. Therefore, placenta previa is not especially worrisome unless it persists beyond the thirtieth week, or the woman bleeds. A placenta that is still blocking the cervix after thirty-two weeks is unlikely to move. Most pregnancies in which placenta previa is diagnosed stay that way after the thirtieth week.

The first episode of bleeding caused by placenta previa is usually light, but it is a warning that must be heeded. The woman must stay on bed rest and abstain from sex for the duration of the pregnancy, unless ultrasound shows that the placenta has moved.

A cesarean section done for a placenta previa may be more complicated than a typical cesarean section. Normally, the placenta detaches from the uterine wall after delivery, and the gaping, huge blood vessels that fed it throughout pregnancy close off when the muscle fibers around them contract. The cervix, however, does not have the same ability to clamp down on the blood vessels so hemorrhaging may occur. The uterus must be closed quickly, and medication may be needed to help the uterus contract well. The practitioner must be prepared to administer blood, if necessary.

Sometimes, placenta previa occurs along with placenta accreta. When that happens, the placenta does not peel away from the uterus normally. It may be stuck to the uterine lining—it may go through the uterine lining into the uterine wall. Placenta accreta is usually accompanied by torrential hemorrhaging, when a skilled obstetrician and transfusions are needed to avoid a disaster. It is usually necessary to do a hysterectomy in such situations.

Placental Abruption

Placental abruption is the tearing away of the placenta from the uterus. While placenta previa causes painless bleeding, placental abruption is accompanied by abdominal pain and uterine contractions. Women are more at risk for placental abruption if they have high blood pressure, had a prior abruption, had an accident where there was a shearing force or blunt trauma to their abdomen, or are cocaine users. Most of the time, though, it occurs in women who have no risk factors. Women who have vaginal bleeding, uterine cramping or pain, and a hard belly before they are due are presumed to have placental abruption.

Tiny abruptions may be hard to diagnose, even with ultrasound.

When a small abruption is suspected, a larger and more catastrophic separation can occur at any time. Practitioners usually try to deliver these babies as soon as is reasonable.

Now that we know what the mother experiences, what happens to the baby when there is a placental abruption? The baby's heart tracing will often show decelerations as it reacts to the loss of its own blood. (The blood loss in placenta previa comes mostly from the mother, while in placental abruption it comes from both mother and baby.) The baby must be delivered quickly once it is clear that a significant portion of the placenta has torn away from the uterus. Labor is continued if a vaginal delivery is imminent. A cesarean section is done if the fetus shows any problems and vaginal birth will take some time.

A final, very rare reason for third-trimester vaginal bleeding is that the fetus ruptures a blood vessel, and the mother discharges some of the baby's blood. Vasa previa involves the umbilical cord inserting into the membrane coming out of the placenta instead of into the placenta itself. Unless one sees bright red blood when the bag of water breaks, and the fetal heartbeat plummets, the chances of this happening are extremely slim.

Incompetent Cervix

Some women have a weak or "incompetent" cervix that prepares for delivery as early as eighteen weeks instead of during the ninth month. This can quickly lead to a preterm birth if it is not treated. When a woman bleeds, she gets a sonogram to make sure that she does not have placenta previa. Her cervix is then examined to see if it is short. If it is, she has what is termed an incompetent cervix. This is remedied by placing a stitch in and around the cervix to secure it and prevent further opening and thinning. This condition and procedure are discussed further in the chapter on premature birth. (See page 209.)

Sometimes, women bleed for reasons that remain unclear even after appropriate testing is done. They can then breathe a sigh of relief and resume their usual activities, bearing in mind that additional bleeding must be reevaluated. Subsequent bleeding may be due to the widening of an initially minute tear of the placenta away from the uterine wall.

Ultrasound is notorious for not detecting small placental abruptions, so any third-trimester bleeding that is not definitely from the cervix must be viewed with caution.

Thus, women should notify their health care provider if they bleed so that they can be evaluated and appropriate interventions (if necessary) can be taken. Two exceptions are: if they have a painless, bloody discharge during the ninth month (caused by cervical changes) or light bleeding after having an internal exam that month.

CHAPTER NINETEEN

Miscarriage

*U*nexpected heavy bleeding, losing the familiar pregnancy symptoms, and/or having an ultrasound that shows no fetal heartbeat can be extremely distressing for an expectant mother. Even though miscarriages are relatively common, few women consider the possibility. If a woman has a miscarriage, she usually experiences a feeling of loss that is accompanied by mourning a child who will never be.

Miscarriage, also called spontaneous abortion, is usually defined as the unintended ending of a pregnancy before the baby could live outside the uterus with medical assistance. (Today, that means before twenty-four weeks' gestation). Ninety-five percent of miscarriages occur during the first trimester, especially during the first nine weeks. Many miscarriages happen before women even know they are pregnant, and they happen much more often than people realize. It has been estimated that as many as one in every three pregnancies ends in miscarriage, and as many as 50 percent of women may have a miscarriage at some point in their lives. The incidence of miscarriage goes up with a woman's age, such that as many as 70 percent of pregnancies in women over forty-one end up miscarrying.

An early miscarriage may actually be happening when a woman finds that her period is a few days late, and then her flow comes heavier than usual.

Because early miscarriages are common, some obstetricians do transvaginal ultrasounds at every pregnant patient's first visit. One out of four sonograms shows signs of a possible problem. Discovering early on that the embryo has died lets the woman come to terms with it before she spends too much time dreaming about, and making plans for, her new baby, and before she has shared good news with too many people. It also allows her to get over the physical aspects of that pregnancy quickly if she decides to have a D and C (dilatation and curettage) soon afterward.

More than 30 percent of women have some vaginal bleeding at the beginning of a pregnancy, but when it is followed by severe uterine cramping, lower abdominal pain, and lower back pain it is likely that she is miscarrying. Until an ultrasound shows that the embryo has died, or a pelvic exam shows that the cervix has dilated, there is always room for hope that the pregnancy will continue. Some women bleed intermittently throughout an entire pregnancy and deliver a healthy, full-term baby.

In the overwhelming majority of early miscarriages, a fetus dies before the body aborts it. That makes it possible to use early ultrasound to predict a miscarriage before the expulsion actually occurs. If it is known that the fetus has died, a woman can choose to wait for a natural abortion to occur or she can schedule a D and C to remove the fetal tissue and uterine lining. A natural abortion can take weeks, while the bleeding that fonlows a D and C usually takes two weeks or less. Women who choose to miscarry normally sometimes experience torrential bleeding that necessitates an emergency D and C. The later in pregnancy the miscarriage occurs, the more likely it is that a D and C will be needed.

Unfortunately, once a miscarriage begins, there is relatively little that can be done to stop it. Doctors often recommend bed rest if the woman is bleeding, but it's unlikely that it makes any real difference. As hard as it is to accept, if it's going to happen, it's going to happen.

Unlike cramping with bleeding, first-trimester cramping without bleeding can be considered perfectly normal. Dehydration or too much activity can cause cramping in the first two trimesters. This can be remedied by drinking fluids and resting. If this doesn't help, or you are in your second trimester, consult your practitioner.

What to Do

A complete miscarriage will cause bleeding that is heavier than a period, with blood clots. Anti-inflammatory drugs like Motrin will help reduce cramping pain. The severe cramping and bleeding get much worse just before the pregnancy tissue is passed. That looks like a beige or gray coccoon, or like a small bubble if it comes early in pregnancy. Try to save this tissue in a jar in a refrigerator, then bring it to the practitioner's office by the next day or so. In early pregnancy (up to ten weeks), unlike normal delivery, the fetus and placenta are usually expelled together. If one is identified, it is assumed that the other was with it, and the miscarriage is complete.

Sometimes heavy bleeding and cramping don't stop, and the pregnancy tissue remains inside. If this continues without slowing down, the practitioner should be called, and an emergency D and C might be needed. If torrential bleeding occurs, where towels instead of large sanitary pads are needed, it is a sign that the body is fruitlessly trying to get rid of pregnancy tissue that is stuck inside the uterus. As long as the tissue sticks to the uterine lining, the uterine muscle can't clamp down on the open blood vessels and stop the bleeding. This usually requires an emergency D and C. Although this may be emotionally traumatic, the bleeding can usually be stopped quickly enough to avoid blood transfusions.

Dilatation and Curettage

The term D and C stands for "dilatation and curettage." The fifteen-minute procedure involves slowly and gently opening the woman's cervix, then scraping out the uterus with a sharp, sterile instrument. It can be done under general or local anesthesia.

Today, suction curettage is done by inserting a plastic tube into the uterus, where it sucks out the contents without scraping the soft lining.

A sharp instrument is inserted afterward to confirm that the uterus is empty.

The cervix is already dilated when an emergency D and C is done on a bleeding woman. When a D and C is done where a spontaneous abortion has not yet started, the cervix must be gently dilated. Some doctors give medication that start the woman bleeding and cramping and make the dilation easier. The suction curettage then follows.

Women may bleed for ten to fourteen days after a D and C. Some women bleed for only a few days, while others bleed off and on until they get their period, about four to six weeks after the procedure. Women should not douche, use tampons, or have intercourse for three weeks after having a D and C, or until all red bleeding ceases, whichever takes longer.

If a woman prefers to avoid a D and C and wait, her chances of having a natural miscarriage are greater if she is less than ten weeks pregnant. If a woman miscarries when she is ten or more weeks pregnant, she is likely to have very heavy bleeding, and her uterus is unlikely to go back to normal without a D and C. This is because the placenta often stays embedded in the uterine lining long after the fetus is expelled.

It was hoped that women with nonviable pregnancies could avoid a D and C by taking drugs that cause abortion. Unfortunately, such medical abortions still don't work too well, and they often end up making the whole process take longer when they fail.

A woman who miscarries needs to know if she has Rh-negative blood. (It could be A-, B-, AB-, or O-.) If she does, and the baby's father has Rh-positive blood, she needs to get an injection of Rhogam within seventy-two hours of the miscarriage's completion. It prevents complications in future Rh-incompatible pregnancies.

Why Miscarriages Occur

Miscarriages occur for many reasons, and the cause in a specific instance is often unknown. The majority occur because the fetus is abnormal. Women often feel guilty about things they think they did that might have caused the pregnancy loss, but those are not usually responsible. One woman thinks it might have been her strenuous exercising and moving heavy boxes. Another attributes it to her having sex early in pregnancy. A third relates it to her prior abortions in college. A forth wonders if it was due to the birth control pills or antihistamines she took before she realized she was pregnant. In reality, women rarely do anything that causes miscarriages. Unless a woman has repetitive miscarriages, there is little reason to search for answers as to why one happened. Some women feel it gives them closure to have the tissue from the D and C sent for genetic analysis to see if there were abnormal chromosomes.

Most women who have one miscarriage have almost the same chance of having a healthy baby as any other mothers. Until they have had up to six miscarriages, women are still likely to have a healthy pregnancy and give birth to a live baby. The mother's age is important, though, as women over forty have higher rates of miscarriage than others, with women forty-two or older miscarrying as much as 70 percent of the time.

A woman has "habitual abortions" if she has two consecutive miscarriages, or three miscarriages interspersed with live births. These women usually get checkups just to make sure that nothing was missed that could help ensure future healthy pregnancies. Even when this is done, it does not usually explain why those miscarriages occurred.

Abnormal Chromosomes

The most frequent reason for a miscarriage is that the embryo had abnormal chromosomes, and this is nature's way of preventing the birth of an abnormal child. At least 60 percent, and possibly more, of miscarriages happen for this reason.

Chromosomes are tiny rodlike structures in the cell that tell it, and the whole organism, how to behave. When the father's sperm and the mother's egg join to create a fertilized egg that becomes an embryo, each parent contributes one set of chromosomes. Sometimes the number or quality of the chromosomes is defective, and a miscarriage results as nature gets rid of a very abnormal embryo. This happens more often with older women than with younger ones because the eggs are older and not as healthy. While men continually produce sperm, it is not until men are in their fifties or older that their sperm has a higher incidence of abnormal chromosomes.

Miscarriages do not usually run in families.

Embryos commonly have abnormal chromosomes for random reasons. Thus, the overwhelming majority of chromosomal abnormalities are not inherited. They occur by chance during the process of fertilization and embryo development. However, in 2 to 5 percent of couples who have had repetitive miscarriages, one partner has abnormal chromosomes that go into every embryo. Couples who have had two or three miscarriages should consider having a blood test by which their chromosomes can be examined for abnormalities. This is called karyotyping.

If a woman has a suction curettage after a fetus dies, the doctor can send some fetal tissue to a genetics lab to see if it had some chromosomal abnormality. This requires having enough fetal cells to grow so that the chromosomes can be looked at through a microscope. If the cells don't grow, nothing can be determined. If the report says that the fetus had abnormal chromosomes, that is assumed to be the reason that the miscarriage occurred. The overwhelming majority of these chromosomally abnormal fetuses simply had "random errors." The rare couple who actually has abnormal chromosomes may want to discuss the implications of this with a genetics counselor.

Uterine Abnormalities

Girls are sometimes born with uterine abnormalities that are called congenital uterine anomalies. When they get pregnant, these abnormalities may cause miscarriage. Since the uterus is a "house" for the growing baby, it must be a structurally sound place that is large enough for a fully grown fetus. If the uterus has an abnormal shape, is too small, or has too little lining, a pregnancy may end in miscarriage.

The most common uterine anomaly is a bicornuate uterus. Instead of the uterus being one united structure, it stays as the two halves that it was in early embryonic life. Bicornuate uteri don't usually cause first-trimester miscarriages. They are more likely to cause preterm labor and delivery, and poor positioning of the baby before delivery. Nevertheless, most women with bicornuate uteri do quite well.

A septate uterus occurs when a piece of tissue separates the uterus into two compartments. The conceptus often can't implant securely or get enough nourishment if it lands on the flimsy tissue. The result may be a miscarriage.

A third congenital abnormality, the T-shaped uterus, occurs almost exclusively in women who were exposed to DES (diethylstilbestrol) when their mothers were pregnant thirty to forty-five years ago. DES is a synthetic, estrogenlike chemical that was prescribed by doctors for women who were thought to be at risk of miscarrying. It was subsequently found that DES caused serious adverse effects in some of those children who are now adults. The youngest of those exposed women with T-shaped uteri will soon be past child-bearing age.

Some uterine abnormalities are acquired, meaning they happen later in life. These include adhesions, polyps, and fibroids. Uterine adhesions are scars in the lining of the uterus. They were usually caused by a D and C, abortion, or surgery to fix congenital uterine abnormalities. Most D and C's don't cause scarring, but if they were done when there was an infection, or after childbirth or abortion, there is a greater chance that scarring occurred. These adhesions can be corrected with a combination of minor surgery and medication.

Fibroids (myomas) are benign growths of the muscle that makes up the uterine wall. They are extremely common and they rarely cause recurrent miscarriages. Most fibroids are assumed to be the cause of recurrent miscarriage only if a miscarriage workup reveals no other problems, the inside of the uterus is greatly distorted by the fibroid, or the fibroids are extremely large. Huge fibroids may force the fetus to share the uterine space. The lack of space eventually causes fetal loss or deformity.

When pregnancy hormones stimulate a fibroid, its rapid growth outstrips the blood supply and it starts to die. That degeneration sometimes results in uterine contractions and miscarriage.

A submucous fibroid may also cause miscarriage. It sits on the inside lining of the uterus, unlike most fibroids, which are in the uterine wall or occasionally attached to the outside of the uterus. A submucous fibroid causes problems early in pregnancy because it is hard for the conceptus to attach itself properly to the fibroid's hard, rubbery surface.

Submucous fibroids can often be removed by minor surgery, unlike other fibroids, which can only be removed by major surgery. When a uterine abnormality is fixed, chances are good that a healthy pregnancy will follow.

Medical Problems

Miscarriages also occur because of medical illness in the mother. Severe or uncontrolled diabetes, lupus, or thyroid problems all increase the chance of miscarriage. Miscarriages result less often from the mother's having genital tract infections or severe heart or kidney disease. Such women should get medical help months before conceiving, in order to improve their health as much as possible first.

Diabetic women greatly improve their chances of having a healthy pregnancy by normalizing their blood sugar through diet and insulin injections as much as possible before getting pregnant. Women with thyroid problems should see an internist or endocrinologist before getting pregnant. Recent research has shown that women with untreated thyroid problems may have children with learning disabilities.

Women who don't have true lupus may produce lupuslike antibodies that may cause miscarriages. This anticardiolipin antibody syndrome can be diagnosed via a blood test when a woman has had recurrent miscarriages or fetal deaths. Women with this syndrome have more stillbirths, severe, early toxemia, and blood clots in their veins than average. Women with this syndrome and recurrent miscarriages should take aspirin and heparin (a blood thinner) injections every day to help maintain their pregnancies. It is thought that these drugs work so well by preventing the clotting of blood vessels that are presumed to otherwise kill the fetus.

Hormonal Causes

Miscarriages may occur in women who do not make enough progesterone. As was discussed earlier, progesterone is the main hormone that the corpus luteum in the ovary makes. The uterus needs the corpus luteum's extra progesterone to keep its lining thick and nurture the conceptus until the placenta takes over at around eleven weeks. A miscarriage may occur if the corpus luteum does not make enough progesterone.

One way to check if a pregnant woman is making enough progesterone is to test her blood. Another way to do it when she is not pregnant is by endometrial biopsy. This samples the woman's uterine lining a few days before she expects her period. A little is suctioned out, then is sent for analysis. (This procedure is uncomfortable for a few seconds, but it doesn't usually require anesthesia.) If the glands of the uterine lining seem immature and underdeveloped for where the woman should be in her cycle, it is assumed that she is not making enough progesterone. This is called a "luteal deficiency," so-named because the corpus luteum isn't doing its job.

If a blood test or biopsy shows that a woman isn't making enough progesterone, she is usually prescribed progesterone. It can be injected, taken in pill form, or inserted as vaginal suppositories. The major side effects of the suppositories are spotting or vaginal itching in some women.

It should be noted that not all practitioners believe that too little progesterone causes miscarriage. They believe that a good progesterone level in early pregnancy can reassure that a good outcome is likely, but a very low level may warn of an impending miscarriage or even an ectopic pregnancy. Giving extra progesterone under these circumstances doesn't help the pregnancy, it only defers the inevitable. It may temporarily stop the woman's bleeding, but it won't prevent miscarriage because the pregnancy wasn't healthy from the start. In such cases, low progesterone was the result, not the cause of the problem. Still, when doctors find a low progesterone level in a pregnant woman, they usually treat it.

Immunologic Problems

Some fertility centers in the United States believe that miscarriages can occur when the parents are too genetically similar to one another. This causes the woman's body to reject the fetus because it thinks the baby is an intruder.

In healthy people, the body's lymphocytes makes antibodies that fight infections caused by intruders such as bacteria or viruses. In order not to mistakenly attack the fetus as a foreign intruder, mothers normally make "blocking antibodies." However, if the baby is too genetically similar to the mother because the father is also similar, the mother will not make blocking antibodies and her body will attack the embryo as if it were a threat. This phenomenon is treated medically by repeatedly injecting the man's white blood cells into the mother in order to blunt her response to the baby.

This treatment is popular among some women because many of them have had healthy babies after using it. Doctors who oppose it believe that these successes occurred by statistical chance, not because that treatment was used. Any woman who has suffered recurrent miscarriage can decide for herself if she wants to try this controversial treatment.

Drugs

Using recreational drugs is harmful, especially during pregnancy when they can cause birth defects. Only cocaine, though, has been clearly linked to miscarriage. It causes blood clots to form behind the placenta, which causes spontaneous abortion.

Ectopic Pregnancies

An ectopic pregnancy is one in which the egg fertilizes in the fallopian tube, then continues to grow outside the uterus instead of where it belongs. Ectopic pregnancies are uncommon in low-risk women. They happen most in women who have had surgery on their fallopian tubes, who already had an ectopic pregnancy, who had pelvic inflammatory disease, or who were exposed to DES in utero.

If an ultrasound shows a pregnancy sac inside the uterus, the risk of a tubal pregnancy is almost zero. (The chance that there is a twin pregnancy, with one in the uterus and the other in the fallopian tube, is one in thirty-thousand.) On the other hand, if a woman with a lot of pregnancy hormone has no such sac detectable on ultrasound, there is a strong likelihood that she has an ectopic pregnancy.

Unlike the uterus, which stretches easily, the fallopian tube is thin-walled and inelastic, and it ruptures quickly when it houses a growing baby. This results in torrential bleeding if it is not diagnosed and treated in time. Surgical treatment for this pulls the ectopic out of the fallopian tube. The tube is removed with the ectopic when the tube is severely damaged, or if the woman does not want to get pregnant again.

Ectopic pregnancy can sometimes be treated medically by giving drugs that dissolve the pregnancy tissue. Surgery is sometimes needed when medication fails to do the job.

Fetal Demise

Fetal demise is the death of a fetus after twenty-four weeks of pregnancy. Like the death of a child, it is one of the worst tragedies that a couple can experience. Fortunately, it happens in less than 1 percent of pregnancies.

Similar to miscarriage, fetal demise can be due to congenital abnormalities or birth defects in the baby, chromosomal abnormalities like Down syndrome or trisomy 13 or 18, or infections such as listeriosis, cytomegalovirus, toxoplasmosis, and fifth disease. Rarely, the umbilical cord may knot or wrap tightly around the baby's neck or a baby may bleed into his mother's, or twin's, bloodstream. At other times, no one knows why a seemingly healthy baby died in the uterus.

Lack of fetal movement is often the first clue that a fetus has died. Women typically feel their babies move for the first time between seventeen and twenty weeks. Later in the pregnancy, a mother should feel these movements every day. If she doesn't, she needs to call her caretaker. (For more on fetal movement, see chapter 17.)

Sometimes fetal death is first noticed when the caretaker can't hear a fetal heartbeat or see the fetal heart beating on a sonogram. When a fetal death occurs, a woman will need a strong support system to help her cope with her loss, discover why the baby died, and decide what next step to take.

About 80 percent of the time, women automatically go into labor within two weeks of the time the baby died. Most women, however, prefer to have labor medically induced. When a miscarriage occurs before twenty-four weeks, a "D and E" (dilatation and extraction) procedure can be done. This removes the baby and the placenta from the uterus.

After twenty-four weeks, a D and E cannot be safely done. The woman must deliver the baby and placenta during normal or induced labor and delivery. One of three possible drugs is used for this. Prostaglandin suppositories may be placed in the vagina every four to six hours until delivery occurs. They may cause the woman to have nausea, vomiting, diarrhea, and fever. Alternatively, Cytotec, a drug that when taken internally treats ulcers, may be placed vaginally to induce delivery. In cases where the cervix is already a little dilated, an intravenous drip of Pitocin may also be used.

Emotional Repercussions

When women miscarry or suffer fetal demise, they (and their husbands) may suffer emotional distress. Losing a hoped-for child so quickly often leaves couples completely unprepared. By the time the fetus has died, the parents have already fantasized a life with their child, and the death of the fetus brings about the death of their dreams. They have wondered what she will look like, how they will feel holding her, what they will name her, and what life with her will be like.

Their emotional pain is sometimes experienced physically, in the form of abdominal pain, headaches, backaches, fatigue, and anxiety, as well as depression. How much upset they feel is usually related to what the pregnancy meant to them, and how well they generally handle adversity.

It is common for women to have stronger emotional responses to miscarriage than their husbands do. The disparity of their reactions can cause marital strain, which compounds the individual suffering of each. Their problems can be heightened when a couple has been having fertility problems or has had repeated miscarriages.

While a caretaker may encourage a couple to try to have another baby as early as two months after a miscarriage, the couple may first have to resolve their fears about having another miscarriage or fetal loss. Since fetal loss can take such an emotional toll on couples, many hospitals now offer support groups for those who have suffered pregnancy loss. The groups may include doctors, psychologists, social workers, nurses, and former patients. Local RESOLVE (RESOLVE's national hotline number is 617-623-0744) and SHARE chapters are also good sources of support.

Most of the grieving for fetal demise occurs within the first year to eighteen months. For first-trimester miscarriages, the period of working through painful feelings tends to be shorter.

Women who suffer fetal demise may want to make changes during subsequent pregnancies. It is not unusual for them to seek a different care provider when that happens. Fortunately, most women who miscarry or who suffer fetal demise will have healthy babies later, although they may need extra emotional support and medical monitoring to help them through.

CHAPTER TWENTY

Premature Birth

A *full-term pregnancy occurs after the thirty-seventh week of pregnancy*, while a premature birth occurs prior to that time. Babies who are born between thirty-four and thirty-seven weeks of gestation have a good long-term prognosis, and their risk of developing significant complications is low. In the short run, they may need temporary help with breathing or oxygenating, but no real problems usually result from that. It is primarily those babies who are born severely premature (between twenty-four and thirty-two weeks of gestation) who may have severe disabilities or even die soon after birth. They account for three-quarters of newborn deaths in the United States.

One of the most devastating, albeit rare complications of prematurity is cerebral palsy. People with cerebral palsy cannot control their movements, they may have speech problems, and they sometimes spend their lives in wheelchairs.

Premature birth occurs for one of two reasons: Doctors occasionally bring it on intentionally in order to save the life of the baby and/or the mother. This may be necessary when the mother develops life-threatening high blood pressure (preeclampsia), when there is fetal distress (a lack of oxygen), when the placenta separates, and the like. This type of labor is called iatrogenic (medically caused) premature labor.

Most preterm births, however, result from spontaneous premature labor. That happens for reasons that are largely unknown, although it is sometimes linked to complications of pregnancy. For example, when the fetal membranes tear prematurely, uterine contractions often start at the same time. That, in turn, leads to premature labor and delivery. When the mother or fetus has an infection, it can also induce labor pains that result in a baby being born long before it is due.

Risk Factors for Prematurity

The most important risk factor for having a premature baby is having already had one or more premature deliveries. A woman who already gave birth prematurely twice has more than a 30 percent chance of doing so again. Other women who are at risk for giving birth prematurely are those with multiple fetuses (twins, triplets, or more), those with too much amniotic fluid, or those who have an abnormally formed uterus (such as unicornuate or bicornuate). Most women, however, who go into preterm labor do not have any risk factors, so it is important for a woman to familiarize herself with the signs and symptoms of preterm labor. They are: constant low back pain, a feeling of pressure in the lower abdomen, vaginal bleeding, and a watery vaginal discharge. Since these symptoms are not very specific, and may also occur in healthy pregnancies, they are most noteworthy if they represent a change for the woman. For example, a sudden increase in vaginal discharge, or a change in the consistency of the discharge, or new abdominal pain, or the start of contractions may all signal preterm labor.

Many women have Braxton Hicks contractions long before they go into labor. These sometimes uncomfortable contractions prepare the uterus for labor. Unlike true labor contractions, they are usually less frequent than every fifteen minutes, they are not regular, and they don't result in the cervix opening up. Women usually describe them as feeling like pressure and discomfort, rather than as painful.

Incompetent Cervix and Cervical Changes

The cervix is the opening of the uterus that leads into the vagina. It provides mechanical support for the fetal membranes during pregnancy. When the cervix is weak or doesn't stay completely closed (incompetent) during pregnancy, or it opens because of uterine contractions, a woman will have preterm labor and delivery.

Preterm labor that results from an incompetent cervix has a different course than that of ordinary premature labor. In the former situation, labor is very abrupt and short, and occurs well before the due date. Typically, the bag of water breaks and the woman delivers shortly thereafter. A woman with ordinary premature labor has a lot of contractions, and internal examinations show a cervix that changes gradually.

The cervix has two parts—the internal os and the external os. When a woman goes into labor, the cervix usually widens and shortens. This can be felt during a pelvic (internal) exam and/or is observable on ultrasound. These cervical changes normally start inside the cervix then move to the outside. This is why early ultrasound signs of cervical change (called funneling, or shortening of the internal os) can give important information about whether or not a woman is likely to go into labor prematurely. These changes can be measured best by a sonogram done by an experienced obstetrical sonographer since the internal os cannot be seen or felt during a manual pelvic exam.

A normal cervix is about one and a half inches or longer. When the cervix is very short, such as less than three-quarters of an inch, the woman is likely to develop preterm labor and should be monitored very closely. If it is caught early, many doctors believe that preterm labor can be successfully treated, at least for some time. Any additional time gained in prolonging the pregnancy is extremely valuable.

A sonogram of the os is done by placing an ultrasound transducer in one of three possible places: on the woman's abdomen, inside her vagina, or on her perineum (the space between the vagina and the pubis).

Placing the transducer on the women's abdomen usually gives an accurate view of the cervix, but the woman needs to have a full bladder when the cervix is viewed. She does this by drinking approximately six to twelve ounces of fluid, then waiting fifteen to thirty minutes without urinating so that her bladder will be full when her cervix is viewed. This can be uncomfortable when a large baby and expanded uterus are already putting pressure on her bladder, but it is not painful.

If the woman's bladder is very stretched, it occasionally makes the cervix look longer than it really is. If the sonographer thinks that the measurement of the cervix through the mother's abdomen wasn't accurate, a second type of sonogram may be done. This is arranged by placing the ultrasound probe in the area of the labia, the folds of skin that surround the vagina. This is called a transperineal sonogram, and can be done without having a full bladder. There are times when even this approach does not allow the cervix to be viewed completely.

A third way to view the cervix is to insert a small, thumb-shaped ultrasound probe into the vagina. Many women have this type of sonogram early in their pregnancies, when the fetus's beating heart first becomes visible. To prepare for a transvaginal sonogram, the woman empties her bladder, then lies on her back on a gynecological table as if she were going to have a regular gynecological exam. A probe is then covered with a sterile, rubber protectant and lubricant and is inserted into her vagina. The entire procedure lasts only about ten minutes. Vaginal sonograms do not cause bleeding, contractions, infections, or harm to the fetus.

Some women have a shorter than normal cervix because they were exposed to diethylstilbestrol (DES) when they were in utero, they are carrying three or more fetuses, they had prior surgery that weakened their cervix, or their cervix was previously torn. Sometimes it is not known why a woman's cervix is unusually short. No matter what the reason, it is important that the cervix stay closed during pregnancy. McDonald circlage, or stitching the cervix shut, has been used for many years to accomplish this. The stitches are usually placed around the eleventh week of pregnancy when a weak cervix is anticipated. The later the stitches are placed, the greater the chance of failure and/or complications such as infection or breaking the amniotic sac. On the other hand, it is not a good idea to put in a stitch much before the end of the first trimester. This is because there is a high incidence of miscarriage anyway during the first trimester, the uterus is much more irritable during this time, and the manipulation required to place the stitch may lead to a miscarriage. When stitches are placed in the cervix, it is usually done in the operating room under spinal or epidural anesthesia. Occasionally, general anesthesia is used. Stitches are then removed in the doctor's office three to four weeks prior to the due date.

Susan was a twenty-six-year-old medical resident who was pregnant with her first baby. She was very excited about being pregnant, but was concerned that it would make it difficult to function at work. She was on call every third night, which meant that she rarely got any sleep at least two nights a week. Every morning, she drank two or three cups of coffee in order to stay awake at hospital rounds.

Thankfully, her pregnancy seemed normal. Susan felt the baby kick for the first time when she was twenty weeks pregnant, at which time she had a comprehensive ultrasound exam at her hospital's high-risk pregnancy unit. Everything seemed fine. Her baby appeared normal, there was a normal amount of amniotic fluid, and her placenta looked healthy.

When Susan was twenty-seven weeks pregnant, she started having low back pain and occasional uterine contractions. She went to her doctor, who found that her cervix was less than an inch long. She was advised to stay home for ten to fourteen days, not to have sex, and to return for a follow-up visit in two weeks.

After spending two days at home, Susan decided to go back to work. Three days later, she thought that she had lost control of her bladder when she wet her panties. She went to the emergency room, where an examination showed that she had "broken her bag of water" (that is, her fetal membranes had ruptured). She was admitted to the hospital, given intravenous fluids, steroids, and antibiotics, and told to stay in bed. Unfortunately, she gave birth two days later to a baby who needed to spend fourteen weeks in an intensive care nursery. Luckily for Susan, the baby was then able to go home, where he recovered nicely after receiving physical therapy.

Three years later, Susan got pregnant again, and she knew that she was at risk for another premature delivery. Her doctor advised her to take it easy from the beginning of the pregnancy. By then, Susan was a doctor in a group practice. She made sure to have a moderate office and hospital schedule and gave up jogging.

Research has shown that strenuous physical activity can lead to higher rates of preterm labor, and that contractions can occur when the mother gets dehydrated for any reason. It is an accepted medical practice for doctors to recommend bed rest for some high-risk patients. In general, we recommend that high-risk patients not jog or do other forms of strenuous exercise, and that all expectant mothers drink enough fluids and avoid getting overheated. Pregnant women who have stressful, physically demanding jobs such as nursing and medical residency are known to have higher rates of preterm labor and other problems. Some women need to put aside the expectation that they can physically punish their bodies and still have healthy pregnancies. Some need to make time to rest and others even need to stop working in order to keep their bodies strong enough to carry through a pregnancy.

All went well during Susan's second pregnancy until she was twenty weeks pregnant. At that point, she again felt ongoing lower back pain and occasional abdominal cramps. She knew that these might be signs of preterm labor and called her doctor. He examined her and told her to go home and stay on "modified bed rest." Modified bed rest involves a woman staying in bed except to take showers, go to the bathroom, and sit down for dinner from time to time.

When Susan was twenty-five weeks pregnant, her abdominal and back pains went away and she was able to resume her usual activities.

Reducing Problems of Prematurity

Women at risk for having premature babies usually want to know what can be done for the baby in the uterus to reduce the problems that it will have after it is born. The major problem of prematurity is called respiratory distress syndrome. That means that the baby does not breathe properly. Since the lungs of premature babies often need more time to develop, their breathing is so shallow that they are unable to get enough oxygen to their vital organs. Too little oxygen leads to other complications, especially in very premature babies. It can result in bleeding in the baby's brain or severe damage to the baby's intestines (called necrotizing enterocolitis, or NEC).

Research has shown that giving the mother steroids can often prevent or reduce respiratory distress. In fact, using steroids to mature the baby's lungs has probably been the most significant advance in fetal medicine during the past ten years. It is also the most frequently used fetal intervention. Steroids not only help the lungs mature, they also decrease other problems that premature babies have, such as necrotizing enterocolitis.

As soon as the baby is born, if it shows any signs of respiratory distress, it is usually given a drug called surfactant, which has dramatically reduced the amount of time such babies must stay in the neonatal intensive care unit. Surfactant enhances the steroid's effect and further improves the condition of the baby's lungs.

Our research group has even given surfactant to babies in utero when premature labor was inevitable. We inserted a surfactant gel through a scope that allowed the medicine to get into the baby's tracheal and bronchial trees. While this procedure is still experimental, it may soon be another advance in fetal medicine.

In Susan's case, her doctor urged her to get steroids to mature the baby's lungs in case he was born prematurely. She agreed. Susan resumed modified bed rest from the time she was twenty-eight weeks pregnant until she was thirty-two weeks pregnant, but she continued to have irregular uterine contractions. She went into labor at thirty-seven weeks of pregnancy and delivered a healthy baby.

Drugs for Preterm Labor

Various drugs are used to treat preterm labor, and each has its benefits and side effects. Magnesium sulfate is the mainstay of such therapy. Unfortunately, there is no good oral form of it so it is usually given through an intravenous pump in the hospital, starting with one dose and followed by a continuous drip. Mothers may initially feel hot flashes or sluggishness, but they usually get used to it. Magnesium sulfate crosses the placenta and may cause short-term sluggishness in the fetus and a decrease in fetal breathing. There has not been any documentation of long-term problems for the baby.

Another group of drugs that is used to stop preterm labor are beta-mimetics. They can be given intravenously, by injections under the skin, or by swallowing. They stop contractions by attaching to special receptors on the smooth muscle of the uterus. The main side effect is the opposite of magnesium sulfate's—it makes women feel jittery, they have trouble sleeping, and their hearts beat faster. Its most severe side effect is pulmonary edema, which causes fluid to build up in the mother's lungs. When the mother is monitored carefully, that very rarely happens, unless she is given beta-mimetics along with magnesium sulfate. That combination increases the likelihood that water will build up in the lungs.

Because beta-mimetics can cross the placenta, they may cause side effects in the baby. The baby's heart beats faster and it also probably feels jittery. While these short-term effects are unpleasant, studies have not found any long-term ill effects of beta-mimetics on the baby.

A third drug, Indocin (indomethacin), is also effective in stopping preterm labor. If it is taken by mouth, it may give the mother an upset stomach, so it is sometimes given as a rectal suppository. It may decrease the amount of amniotic fluid surrounding the baby. Women who get Indocin should be monitored sonographically by a specialist in high-risk pregnancy. There need to be frequent checks of the amount of amniotic fluid. If problems with the amniotic fluid develop, Indocin is discontinued and the side effects usually disappear within twelve hours.

Some time later, Susan told her doctor that she wanted to have a third child. She wanted to know about new developments in the area of preterm labor diagnosis and treatment, and there was potentially promising news to give her. It was discovered that the placenta makes a biochemical substance called fibronectin. Mothers who are about to go into preterm labor make extra amounts of it. It is detected by putting a cotton swab into the vagina and measuring the amount of fibronectin in the vaginal secretions. An abnormally high amount means the mother is at risk for preterm labor. Unfortunately, further research is needed to see if the amounts of fibronectin detected this way will reliably predict preterm labor. In sum, there is much a woman and her doctor can do to prevent preterm labor. If a woman knows that she is at risk, and she follows her doctor's advice, she has a good chance of having a full-term baby, or of having a healthy baby when prematurity is inevitable.

Premature Rupture of Membranes (PROM)

The fetus lies inside fluid in a thin, stretchy amniotic membrane. Together with the cervix and mucus plug, it keeps bacteria from getting inside the amniotic bag, or "sac," via the vagina. Once the amniotic sac ruptures, there is no longer a barrier to bacteria, and the risk of a fetal infection increases. This is why doctors "start the clock ticking" once the bag of water breaks, and induction or cesarean section are planned if labor doesn't follow soon thereafter.

On the other hand, the bag of water can break long before the baby is due, in which case the risk of significant prematurity far outweighs the risk of infection. Fortunately, this type of rupture of membranes long before the due date does not happen often. When it does, it is sometimes because an infection produced chemicals that caused the bag of water to break. When this is not the case, rather than inducing labor, the doctor keeps the woman under close watch and gives her blood tests and sonograms. He or she intervenes only when there are signs of infection, when there is so little fluid that the baby is threatened, or when the baby reaches maturity.

Steroids are often given when the membranes rupture so early that the baby needs it to mature his lungs, while labor is forestalled for those forty-eight hours by giving the mother a uterine-relaxing medication.

When premature rupture of membranes occurs close to maturity, and contractions do not follow, practitioners induce labor within twenty-four to forty-eight hours. Induction should be done sooner if the woman has group B strep. In any event, when the bag of water breaks, the woman should notify her health care practitioner, who will know what to do.

When the bag of water breaks before twenty-four weeks, an extremely rare occurrence, the baby is not yet viable outside of the uterus. Since a bad infection could harm the mother and her fetus, the standard response offered is to terminate the pregnancy. The woman is counseled about the baby's prognosis if he will be born during the next few weeks, the risks of infection, and the effects that too little amniotic fluid will have on the fetus since the lungs need the fluid to develop properly. If she wants, the doctor can help her keep the pregnancy nonetheless.

How does a woman know when her bag of water has broken? There is a sudden loss of fluid from the vagina, similar to what it feels like to lose control of one's bladder. Since women toward the end of pregnancy sometimes lose control of their bladders, they may not know what type of fluid is coming out. The flow of fluid after breaking the bag of water, unlike urination, does not end after a few seconds. The fluid continues to trickle or leak. If a woman puts on a sanitary pad, it will get wet. The important point is not how much fluid there is over a few minutes but whether or not the trickle continues. If the woman coughs or moves abruptly, there may be a small gush of fluid in response.

Sometimes all a woman sees is vaginal "bleeding." If the fluid is very watery and more pink than red, it is likely to be amniotic fluid with a few red blood cells from the cervix mixed in. A drop of blood in a lot of water can look like a lot of blood.

If a woman is in doubt as to whether or not her bag of water has broken, she should call her practitioner. The practitioner can insert a speculum into the vagina and see if there is a pooling of fluid. A bit of this fluid is removed, or the vagina and cervix are swiped if there is no fluid, and a piece of special paper is dipped into it to see if it is the same alkalinity as amniotic fluid. If this doesn't give a clear answer, the fluid can be examined under a microscope to see if it has the unique features of amniotic fluid. Usually, however, the diagnosis is obvious. Anything that is mucuslike, or so insignificant that a pad is not needed, is generally not amniotic fluid.

Delivery of Premature Babies

Cesarean section is done more often with preterm births than with term babies. This is because preterm babies are much more likely to be in an unusual position for delivery, such as breech or transverse. Since their heads are disproportionately large for their bodies, a cesarean section is considered to be a safer way to deliver them if they are breech. Also, preterm babies are weaker than full-term, so when there is fetal distress doctors resort to cesarean section more readily. This is because premature babies have less strength to withstand the stress of labor, and bleed into their brains more easily than full-term babies do. Finally, since premature babies have a higher incidence of brain impairment than full-term babies, doctors may want to limit their legal risk by avoiding a difficult labor and delivery.

Preterm birth is responsible for a large percentage of neonatal death and disability. Lowering the incidence of preterm birth will improve our babies' health and reduce the number of babies in neonatal intensive care units.

PART III

Labor and Delivery

CHAPTER TWENTY-ONE

The Big Day

At the beginning of the ninth month, practitioners start checking the woman to see if the body has started preparing for labor and delivery. A baby can be in one of three positions before delivery—head-down, bottom-down (breech), or transverse (sideways). The cervix can be open or closed, soft or firm, long or short. When it is soft, open, and short, delivery is at hand.

The Baby's Position

A baby needs to be head-down or buttocks-down in order to be delivered vaginally. When a baby's head is against the cervix in the usual downward position for birth, it automatically blocks the umbilical cord from exiting. This is the safest position for delivery.

If a baby is transverse, or lying sideways, he cannot be delivered vaginally. A woman who goes into labor that way has a higher risk of cord prolapse, an unusual situation where the umbilical cord stops floating freely in the uterus, drops through the cervix, and gets its blood supply cut off. This causes an emergency necessitating an immediate cesarean section. A transverse baby can also get stuck inside the uterus so that he is hard to extract, even via cesarean section.

A breech baby is one whose feet or buttocks are against the cervix. They are also more likely to have a cord prolapse, especially when the feet present first. Breech or transverse babies may be rotated into a better position by external version.

External Version

In external version, the woman lies on her back while expert hands manipulate the baby externally into the right position using ultrasound as a guide. If she is having contractions, some practitioners give her medications to relax her uterus. This makes it easier to move the baby, who is not forced. The person moving the baby can feel if there is give, and if the baby is moving readily or not.

External version by an experienced practitioner involves a miniscule risk of tearing the placenta away from the wall, or of causing a cord accident.

External versions are not always successful. If the baby remains transverse close to the due date, a cesarean section is scheduled.

Delivering Breech Babies

Breech babies may present a complicated set of delivery decisions because of their potential problems: Rarely, a breech baby's body slips through the cervix while the head stays trapped in the uterus, unable to budge. An arm may also get hooked around his head and not be deliverable without persistent pulling that injures a nerve. Although these complications are rare, few obstetricians today are willing to deliver breech babies vaginally because of the prevalence of lawsuits during the past twenty years. The result is that breech babies are typically delivered by cesarean section, especially if they are a woman's first.

If the woman and practitioner want to attempt a vaginal breech delivery, an ultrasound should be done to make sure that the baby's head is flexed and not extended, and that the baby is not too large. Most obstetricians will only do it then if the woman has previously delivered a baby vaginally and this baby is "frank breech," meaning his legs are near his face and his buttocks are near the cervix. A prior vaginal delivery tells the doctor that the woman's pelvis is large enough for the task at hand. Many studies have shown that when babies are not the woman's first, their rumps are against the cervix, the legs are toward the top of the uterus, and the chin is down, they do as well whether they are delivered vaginally or by cesarean section.

Early Labor

When the internal examination at or beyond thirty-six weeks shows the cervix is closed, long, and firm, labor is probably still some time away. When the cervix is open (dilated), short, and soft, labor may be close at hand.

When early (prodromal) labor begins, contractions are brief, mild, tolerable, and irregular. They might continue for hours, even become more regular, then die out. As long as the baby is moving normally, there is no need for the low-risk woman to notify or be checked by her practitioner. Such labor is unlikely to have progressed much, and it is difficult to know when more intense labor will start. Some women can even have this type of labor for several days. If it goes on for too long, the laboring woman might feel exhausted and need to be admitted for intravenous medication or be stimulated with Pitocin to get the labor to progress. In general, though, women should try to ride these contractions out until the labor pains get stronger.

A woman having her first baby should call her caretaker and prepare to leave for the hospital when contractions occur every four to five minutes for an hour, each lasting forty-five seconds or more, and are so uncomfortable that she can't talk or do much else during a contraction. If she is already feeling the need to bear down, she needs to get to the hospital quickly.

A woman who has previously given birth tends to have a shorter labor than one giving birth for the first time. Some women who have already had children may be far along in labor without having felt strong contractions. The physical reward of having previously given birth is the easier delivery of subsequent babies. The pelvic bones and abdominal muscles have already accommodated a child, and the cervix and vagina have already been "conditioned" to allow a baby to pass through.

On the other hand, a woman who has had many prior babies may find that her uterine contractions are no longer as strong as they once were because the uterine muscles have been so stretched by many pregnancies.

Once a woman's bag of water breaks, she is evaluated to make sure that is what happened. The baby is checked to see if he or she is still head-down and doing well. A good fetal heart rate shows that the umbilical cord is not getting squeezed and that the baby is not stressed. The water should be clear and not be stained with fetal bowel movement (meconium). When the amniotic fluid is green or yellow, the baby may be in trouble.

Meconium

Normally, a baby evacuates its bowels some time after birth. Sometimes, however, it does it into the amniotic fluid that surrounds it while still in the uterus. The fetus, especially under stress, may then swallow the contaminated fluid into its lungs. That can make the baby sick. Meconium in the amniotic fluid becomes more common in babies that are postdue. This is one reason why a pregnancy is almost never allowed to continue beyond the forty-second week.

When a baby is born with meconium, the pediatrician may put a laryngoscope down the baby's throat in order to suction out the meconium from the windpipe before it gets breathed into the lungs. It is best to do this before the baby has started taking breaths. Since the baby cannot cry with this instrument down its throat, it sometimes goes limp. While this frightens parents, they shouldn't worry. The baby will start crying and turn pink once it is stimulated.

Progression of Labor

Once the woman goes into labor, she should notify her labor coach. That might be her husband, her mother, a sister, a close friend, or even a hired professional labor coach known as a doula. That person should be emotionally supportive, as well as make the mother as comfortable and effective as possible as she labors and delivers. Of course her labor coach accompanies the woman to the hospital.

Once a woman goes to the labor suite, her blood pressure and temperature are checked. She is examined internally to see how much her cervix has opened, then the baby's heart rate and the frequency and duration (not intensity) of her contractions are checked. Labor may continue for many hours until the cervix is four to five centimeters dilated. In fact, this latent phase of labor is not considered to be unduly long unless it takes more than twenty hours for a first baby or fourteen hours for subsequent ones.

As a rule, once a first-time mother's cervix is five centimeters dilated and thin during active labor, it will dilate one centimeter or more every hour until the cervix is fully open (ten centimeters). If an hour passes and the cervix has not dilated an additional centimeter, the practitioner may give Pitocin.

Pushing

The second stage of labor is when the woman pushes the baby out. It begins when the cervix is ten centimeters wide, and it ends with the baby's delivery. The first-time mother may need to push for two hours or more, while a woman having her second baby may need to do so for only fifteen minutes, with tremendous variation. The position from which the woman pushes best also varies from person to person, and may change as the baby moves.

Laboring women push the same way they would expel a bowel movement. They should not feel self-conscious about what else they expel along with the baby. One popular way of doing this is to take a "cleansing" breath as the contraction starts, then take a deep breath and hold it for a count of ten while pushing into one's bottom. Then exhale and begin the cycle again.

Here is a common way to push when you are lying in bed or on a delivery table. Keep your head and shoulders raised and knees bent. Relax your perineum, then breathe deeply in and out. Hold onto the backs of your thighs while pushing with your knees spread wide apart. Take a deep breath in, hold it, and push for ten seconds. Exhale. Breathe in deeply again and hold it while you push for ten seconds. Exhale. Repeat a third time. Take a deep breath and relax until the next contraction. Push only with the contractions. Do this on your back or on one side or the other, depending upon the baby's position and how you push best. Some women (approximately 10–15 percent) experience shivering during labor. This is not cause for concern as it is due to active muscle work.

Monitoring the Baby during Labor

To imagine what labor contractions might feel like to a baby, think of small earthquakes surrounding you every two or three minutes. This is why obstetricians, perinatologists, and medical researchers all agree that the baby should be carefully watched to try to avoid any problems that can occur during labor. The main way this is done is by measuring the fetal heart rate.

A practitioner will look at several measures to assess whether or not a baby's heart is beating normally: First, are there between 120 and 160 heartbeats a minute? If so, that is a good sign. A heart rate above 160 is too fast (tachycardia), and below 110 is too slow (bradycardia).

Next, the caretaker will see if the baby is showing normal heart rate variability. A heart rate is not supposed to stay exactly the same over time. For example, it may be 130 beats per minute for a few seconds, then 137 for a few seconds, then 128 for a few seconds, and so on.

When a baby is not getting enough oxygen, the heart rate does stay the same, and its tracing on a graph looks like a straight line instead of a series of small ups and downs. Or the baby's heart rate may swing wildly from beat to beat, with the tracing jumping up and down in a short, spiky pattern.

Finally, the caretaker looks for healthy changes in the fetal heart rate. Accelerations (speeding up) and decelerations (slowing down) in heart rate are monitored. There are usually decelerations in the fetal heart rate during labor, and they typically occur in three ways:

Each time the uterus starts a contraction, less blood flows to the baby through the placenta, and the baby's heart rate slows at the same time. This is an early deceleration, so-called because the drop in heart rate occurs early in the contraction. This is believed to occur because the baby's head is squeezed during each contraction. This type of slowed heart rate is considered normal. Such uterine stress may be challenging but not threatening for a healthy fetus. In other words it is stressed, not distressed.

Variable decelerations can occur at any time—before, during, or even after a contraction. Variable decelerations are the most common type of fetal heart slowing. They are believed to be caused when the umbilical cord is squeezed by the baby or is squeezed between the baby and the uterus. Some umbilical cord compression during labor is common, and babies usually adapt well to normal variable decelerations. On the other hand, very deep, recurrent, variable decelerations may stress the baby. When that happens, the practitioner watches the tracings closely and tries to improve the situation.

The third type of fetal heart slowing occurs during late decelerations. They are called "late" because they happen after the uterine contraction is under way. Late decelerations may signal that the baby is having trouble. It is believed that late decelerations start when the baby has little oxygen in reserve and its heart can no longer react promptly to the stress of labor. Having one or two late decelerations doesn't mean that the baby is in immediate danger or that the mother needs an emergency delivery. It does, however, usually mean that the baby needs more oxygen and continual checking.

A fetal heart tracing that shows a heart rate staying above 160 (tachycardia) may be due to a number of worrisome reasons: The baby may not be getting enough oxygen; it may have anemia or an infection. The mother may be dehydrated or have a fever. It could even be a prolonged acceleration that will eventually go back to normal. This is why the mother gets fluids through an intravenous line, her temperature and pulse are checked, and a blood test is done to see if she has an infection when the initial monitoring shows fetal tachycardia.

The best way we know of getting more oxygen to the baby is to give it to the mother through a breathing mask. The mother's position is often changed by moving her onto her right or left side, and she is given more fluids. If the fetal distress is caused by contractions that are too frequent or too intense, the mother may get medication to relax her uterus.

If Pitocin is causing too-frequent contractions, it is turned off. These measures usually reduce the fetus's distress significantly because they increase its oxygen supply.

If the fetal heart rate pattern is not reassuring, a fetal scalp sample may be done to see if the baby is okay. The doctor does this by inserting a specially designed blade through the vagina and minutely nicking the baby's scalp. A few drops of blood are removed and sent to the lab to see if the baby is getting enough oxygen. The test results usually take but a few minutes to get back. If they show that the baby is in trouble, he is delivered quickly.

An urgent delivery is also necessary when the above-mentioned measures are not effective and the fetal heart decelerations continue. If the woman's cervix is fully dilated, and the baby is close to delivering, a forceps or vacuum extraction delivery is often done. Both are safe procedures when done by a well-trained, skilled doctor. Otherwise, a cesarean section must be done.

One can now see why obstetrical caretakers don't agree about whether continually monitoring the baby's heart rate is helpful. Those who prefer it have watched mothers enter labor with seemingly healthy babies who were not carefully monitored and who ended up stillborn. Also, continuous monitoring is more objective and depends less on having someone check it periodically. This is advantageous when a delivery suite is very busy or when skilled nurses are not readily available.

Some practitioners believe that periodically listening to the fetal heart rate is as good as doing so continuously, even though periodic monitoring has not been carefully studied. Those who oppose continuous fetal monitoring know that it increases the chance that the mother will get an unnecessary cesarean section when the monitoring shows potentially ominous, albeit actually harmless, information.

Should women then have continuous or intermittent fetal heart rate monitoring? We believe that every high-risk mother should have her baby continuously monitored during labor and delivery. The same holds true for women with meconium-stained amniotic fluid, too little amniotic fluid, or those whose initial fetal heart tracing in the labor suite shows decelerations. Other mothers should decide for or against continual fetal monitoring via a dialogue with their caretaker.

When should monitoring occur? When active labor begins. If continuous fetal monitoring isn't used, the baby may be monitored every half hour if the heart rate remains stable during contractions, or after every contraction when the mother is pushing.

External and Internal Monitors

There are two possible kinds of fetal heart monitor to use—external or internal. An external monitor secures a belt with two small transducers on it to the woman's belly. One transducer is an ultrasound probe like the one used during a non-stress test. The other transducer measures the frequency and intensity of the uterine contractions. Once the transducers are attached, the woman can't move much, and even changing positions while lying down can displace the belt and disrupt the monitor. Some women find the resulting confinement uncomfortable, but the monitoring is not painful.

Once the amniotic sac membranes rupture when the "waters break," an internal monitor can be used. This involves inserting a small electrode into the vagina and corkscrewing it superficially into the baby's scalp via a tiny wire. This usually causes little discomfort for the mother. In our experience, having monitored more than ten thousand babies, we rarely saw any problems affecting the baby using either type of monitoring. There were only two instances of scalp infection due to internal monitoring, and both were treated successfully. When there are any questions about the fetal heart rate, it may be prudent to use the more precise internal monitor.

Let's see how the above information is actually applied. Jenny was a twenty-two-year-old woman having her first baby after a healthy pregnancy with no medical problems. When she came to the hospital in labor, the doctor did a pelvic exam and found that her cervix was three to four centimeters dilated. The baby's head was touching the cervix and the amniotic sac had not yet broken. The doctor listened to the baby's heart using a portable Doppler monitor and found it to be normal.

Jenny believed that walking between contractions would speed up her labor, and we encouraged her to do so. She did this for the next two and a half hours, until it became difficult for her to bear the pain of her contractions. At that time, we reexamined her and found her cervix to be five to six centimeters dilated. This showed good labor progress.

She was then placed on an external fetal monitor. It showed a stable fetal heart rate, with a normal base rate of 140 beats per minute. It also showed variable decelerations. The most common cause of this is the cord looping around the baby's neck.

We tried to get the decelerations to lessen by moving the mother onto her right side, then left side, but it didn't work. The variable decelerations not only continued, they got deeper and lasted longer. We then did an amnioinfusion where we injected a weak, sterile solution of salt in water into the uterus through a small plastic tube. Warm saline must be used because injecting cold fluid will cause the baby and mother to shiver. This fluid then filled the uterus so that the baby had more room to swim, and the umbilical cord, with its three blood vessels, floated. This well-accepted procedure has few complications.

The baby's variable decelerations stopped twenty minutes after Jenny got the fluid. She later delivered a healthy baby boy with a loop of umbilical cord around his neck. The loop was removed as soon as his head was delivered.

Sarita was a thirty-six-year-old mother of three children. All of her pregnancies and deliveries had been normal and uneventful. When she went into active labor with her fourth baby, she came to the hospital. Her blood pressure and heart rate were normal. She had such painful contractions every three to four minutes that it was hard to lie still. When she was examined internally, her cervix was three to four centimeters open and her water had not yet broken. The baby's heart rate was then measured at 120 beats per minute, but with less than normal variability. The doctor discussed with her and her husband the fact that the external monitoring was not reassuring. The couple agreed to have the doctor internally monitor the baby. That required breaking the amniotic sac.

When that happened, there was only a small amount of fluid. The doctor then placed a spiral electrode on the baby's head and watched the monitor tracing for the next fifteen minutes. It showed a flat line with periodic changes that suggested late decelerations.

When a baby shows late decelerations, the most important question to ask is "Is the baby getting enough oxygen?" One way of finding out is to test the acidity of the baby's scalp by doing a scalp pH test. A normal pH is above 7.20. If the scalp pH is normal, labor is allowed to proceed. If the scalp pH is low, the baby is getting too little oxygen, and action needs to be taken.

In Sarita's case, it took only five minutes to get the results of her baby's scalp pH. It was below normal (7.15). Sarita's doctor recommended that she have an immediate cesarean section.

Sarita's son was delivered with an entire neonatal team present (these are pediatric specialists who care for newborn babies). The boy had an Apgar score of 5 at one minute, and 8 at five minutes. (See page 235.) He was given extra oxygen as soon as he was born, and was later transferred to a neonatal unit for observation. He did well and was discharged from the hospital four days later. He is now a healthy seven-year-old.

Episiotomy

Once the mother is in the second stage of labor, the baby's head is squeezed through the birth canal. When the crown emerges, the practitioner must decide if the perineum is stretching nicely or not. If it is, an attempt is usually made to deliver the baby without doing an episiotomy—surgically cutting the floor of the vagina. A stretched perineum that is not cut may tear. Women whose babies have fetal distress or who have thick meconium are more likely to need episiotomies. Time is of the essence, and one cannot wait the extra minutes that it takes to deliver a baby over an intact perineum. A woman with a very large baby may also need an episiotomy to avoid difficulty delivering the baby's shoulders.

There are two basic kinds of episiotomies: One is cut from the back of the vagina toward the anus (midline episiotomy), while the other is cut diagonally from the back of the vagina toward the right buttock (right mediolateral episiotomy). The first heals more easily, but is also more likely to extend all the way into the rectum during a difficult delivery. Such a tear is called a fourth-degree laceration and must be repaired very carefully. While healing, the woman must make sure to keep her stools soft, using stool softener if necessary, and not use an enema or rectal suppository for six weeks.

Birth

Usually, once the baby's head comes out, a little pushing, gentle leverage and sliding causes one shoulder to come out, then the other, then the rest of the body.

Many doctors use forceps and vacuums as an alternative to cesarean sections when possible. Many times, a baby's head is so low that it is more traumatic to pull it through a cesarean section cut than to use a pair of forceps or pull it gently with a vacuum cup attached to the head. In well-trained, experienced hands forceps and vacuum are extremely useful and carry little risk relative to the alternatives. Forceps got a bad reputation years ago when very high forceps were used to pull out babies whether or not the uterus had enough room to do so.

Today, strict criteria are followed as to when to use forceps. When forceps are used, babies may be born with red or mildly bruised cheekbones but these marks disappear quickly.

Vacuum cups were once made out of a rigid material that caused scalp lacerations. Today's silastic cups are so soft that injury is rare, (see fig. 5a and 5b), although they do leave a scalp swelling under the area where they were placed. This "chignon" usually disappears in a day or two. Once the baby is out, the father may be offered scissors with which to cut the umbilical cord. The practitioner will do the cutting herself if the father doesn't want to; if the cord is wrapped around the baby's neck and needs to be cut before the baby's shoulders are delivered; or if there is thick meconium or fetal distress, and time is of the essence.

The baby is dried, someone suctions his nose and throat to get out the secretions and amniotic fluid, then an Apgar score is given. Apgar scores were developed by Dr. Virginia Apgar solely to guide pediatricians as to when a baby might need help breathing. Despite popular misconception, there is little relationship between Apgar scores and a child's intelligence or success.

Apgar scores are given to babies at one minute and five minutes af-

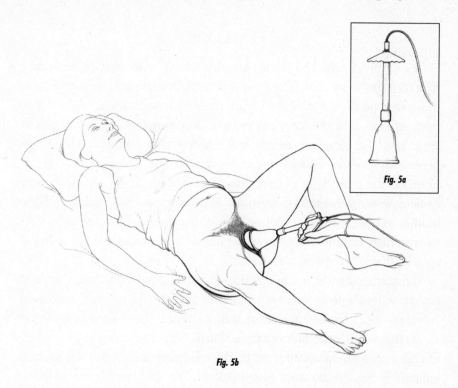

Fig. 5a

Fig. 5b

ter birth. Zero, one, or two points are given for each of five items: color, heart rate, muscle tone, breathing, and movements. A score of 7 or higher is fine. Babies rarely get a 10, because almost no newborns are pink all the way into their fingertips and toes. It is normal that their circulation hasn't yet reached the ends of their extremities.

	Tone	Color	Cry	Heart Rate	Respiration	TOTAL
			Apgar Chart			
1 minute	2	1	2	2	2	9
5 minutes	2	2	2	2	2	10

Cord Blood Donation

Cord blood, which is really placental blood, is an amazing substance that contains stem cells. These are special cells that give rise to the three important parts of a person's blood: the white cells, which fight infection, the red cells, which carry oxygen and nutrients to the body's organs, and the platelets, which make blood clot. People with certain genetic diseases or leukemia can be deficient in these blood components. Until recently, a person with leukemia might get chemotherapy to destroy the cancerous cells in his bone marrow, then receive a bone marrow transplant from a donor. Hopefully, the transplanted cells start to replenish the patient's diseased marrow and produce healthy blood cells.

Unfortunately, it is often hard to find a compatible bone marrow donor, unless a close relative's matches exactly. Since 1993, placental blood has been banked and these stem cells have been used in some patients instead of bone marrow transplants.

The cord blood is collected in the following way: After the umbilical cord is cut, the part that is still attached to the placenta is drained to provide two ounces or more of blood. The blood is then typed and stored. Unlike bone marrow transplants, collecting cord blood is painless to the donor, it is richer than bone marrow in stem cells, and it doesn't require an exact match to the recipient.

A number of private blood banks are now pitching expectant women about the need to bank their cord blood in case it's needed to save the life of a loved one. Thousands of women have already paid about $1,500 for the initial donation, and about $100 a year for storage of the frozen blood. Does this really make sense?

The answer is probably no. There is almost no chance that this blood will ever be used. Why? Cord blood is rarely used unless one has a familial genetic disease that requires a bone marrow transplant. If there is such a disease, there are blood banks that will provide this service for free.

In fact, doctors dissuade storing one's own baby's blood for familial use unless there is a genetic disease in the family. That is because it puts those units out of reach for others who might actually need it. Also, if a baby develops leukemia, some think that as much as 50 percent of the time some cancer cells may be present at birth. That blood would not be recommended for transplant purposes.

Another benefit of donating only to public blood banks is that they make sure that the blood does not contain infectious diseases or genetic blood problems. So, if you are inclined to donate cord blood, please contact your local blood bank.

Unexpectedly Rapid Delivery

We've all heard stories about women who gave birth on a bus or in a taxi or a car on the way to the hospital. If a woman ever feels like the baby is coming out and no medical personnel are nearby, she should call 911 for an ambulance. Then she should lie against her back with her knees bent and spread as far apart as possible and just let the baby come. If someone is with her, he or she should simply guide the baby out, preferably onto something clean and soft. Don't try to hold the baby back by closing the mother's legs or holding a hand over the baby's head to prevent its exit. Don't worry about cutting the umbilical cord. The blood flow to the cord will stop on its own and the cord can be cut later.

Induced Labor

There are times when practitioners cause labor to occur instead of waiting for it to happen spontaneously. This is known as induced labor. Some induced labor is scheduled well in advance, while other times it is a decision made close to the due date. Some reasons why labor may be induced include:

1. The baby is overdue. Induction is recommended when the baby is already two or more weeks late since the risk to the fetus climbs precipitously after forty-two weeks. If a non-stress test and biophysical profile show problems such as too little amniotic fluid at forty-one weeks, induction is recommended.

2. The membranes have ruptured prematurely. If labor doesn't start after the bag of water has broken, labor will be induced. The longer it

takes between the breaking of water and delivery of the baby, the greater the risk of infection to mother and child. Some practitioners induce labor almost immediately after premature rupture of membranes.

3. Nonmedical reasons: A woman may be far away from her practitioner and spontaneous labor may mean that she might deliver before reaching the hospital. Some women want induced labor to avoid delivering during inconvenient times. If inductions are done due to nonmedical considerations, the cervix should be ripe and ready or problems could result.

4. The fetus has problems. Labor is induced when the fetus is not doing well. For example, delivery is expedited if the fetus has stopped growing because he is not getting enough nutrition or oxygen, or if he has become extremely anemic due to Rh problems.

5. The mother may be high risk. Women with high blood pressure, diabetes, or kidney disease may have placentas that deteriorate too early near the end of pregnancy. These pregnancies are ended early by induction if they don't end spontaneously first.

6. The woman is toxemic. Induction is necessary when toxemia occurs close to the due date.

7. The fetus has died. Grief counselors usually advise pushing off delivery of a dead fetus until after fetal death has been confirmed, although most patients in our experience prefer to be delivered immediately. In either case, labor is induced.

8. The uterus is infected. When this happens, delivery needs to occur soon. If induced labor will take too long, a cesarean section is done.

How Labor Is Induced

The cervix needs to be ripened before labor can be induced. When that hasn't already occurred, the woman comes to the hospital and the practitioner puts a prostaglandin gel or similar substance deep in the vagina. It stays there for hours.

This gel sometimes does nothing for hours; at other times it results in contractions. Cervodil is a ribbon soaked with prostaglandins and it releases them slowly. It takes more time than the gel, but it can be removed if there are too many contractions. Cytotec, an oral medication usually used to heal ulcers, is also effective at ripening the cervix and inducing labor. While the company that makes Cytotec recommends not using it to induce live births, that will probably change since the drug has proved itself invaluable in ripening the cervix.

If the cervix is already somewhat open, short, and soft, it shows that enzymes have started breaking down the firm substance that makes up the cervix. This makes induction easier, and only Pitocin needs to be given.

Pitocin is the commercially prepared form of oxytocin, the chemical that a woman's body makes to start labor. The woman gets hooked up to a pump that gives drops of Pitocin through an intravenous line instead of waiting for the woman to make enough oxytocin of her own. If Pitocin causes too many contractions, the pump is turned off, and the contractions stop quickly. Pitocin is also given to stimulate a labor already in progress if the contractions have died out, no progress is made in a reasonable amount of time, or an epidural has relaxed the uterus so it doesn't contract.

Pitocin got a bad reputation a half century ago when it was given without careful calibration, sometimes causing too many contractions at once, fetal distress, and rarely, uterine rupture. Pitocin must still be used cautiously with women whose uteri have been stretched more than normal, such as with full-term twins or when there is too much amniotic fluid; when a woman is having a vaginal delivery after a prior cesarean section; or when she has already given birth to many children, because it may lead to uterine rupture or heavy bleeding after delivery.

Labor may also be stimulated by breaking the bag of water. Tearing the membranes releases prostaglandins, which stimulate labor. Prostaglandins, in turn, cause enzymes to be made which soften the cervix. While breaking the bag of water alone sometimes initiates labor, practitioners usually give a little Pitocin at the same time.

Some doctors insert their fingers through the ripe cervix and sweep them around in order to release prostaglandins that will start labor. Unfortunately, this often does little more than cause bleeding and cramping.

Women with a ripe cervix have often heard that there are things they can do to bring on labor. Walking and physical activity is fairly useless, eating certain foods doesn't help, and having sex is debatable, at best. Women have traditionally drunk two ounces of castor oil in a glass of orange juice. It causes abdominal cramping and diarrhea, which sometimes leads to labor. At other times, it only keeps women on the toilet with profuse loose bowel movements.

Some women want induced labor if the baby is becoming very large to reduce the chance of needing a cesarean section. Studies have shown that inducing labor under these circumstances does not reduce the cesarean section rate, even though the baby may be half a pound or a pound smaller. Something about natural labor balances out any advantage of having an induced smaller baby. While it would be reasonable to induce if the woman's cervix is already very ripe, it is best to leave matters to nature if the cervix is closed, long, or firm and the baby's head hasn't yet dropped.

It seems that induced labor is more painful than spontaneous labor based on the fact that epidural anesthesia is much more necessary in the former situation. Also, induced labor requires a woman to lie in bed with intravenous lines and monitors, with little ability to move around. While some women plan to have a natural, unanesthetized labor, almost every induced woman counts her blessings that anesthesia was available!

The day that a woman gives birth is one of the most memorable and wondrous days of her life. The better prepared she is for the challenges that she might face, the less likely that she will have negative associations to labor and delivery. Childbirth preparation classes are invaluable because they give women and their birth attendants a preview of what lies ahead, thereby reducing much of the anxiety that might otherwise occur.

CHAPTER TWENTY-TWO

Anesthesia during Labor

It is hard for a woman to know how she will feel during labor and de- livery. Every labor is different, and it is especially hard for first-time mothers to anticipate what labor will feel like when it progresses in earnest. The first stage of labor may have some labor pains that feel like strong menstrual cramps. When pushing begins, they might feel intense pressure on the rectum, followed by a burning, tearing sensation at the perineum. "Back labor" is almost intolerable flashes of pain that come from the lower back. They have been likened to the feeling of passing kidney stones. It is a rare woman who has so little pain in labor that the baby naturally delivers with minimal discomfort.

There are a variety of techniques and philosophies as to how best to go through labor. Lamaze, one of the natural methods, encourages women to focus on something other than the pain. It also teaches how to breathe during contractions and relax between them. The Bradley method encourages women to vocalize and move with their pain, much as a surfer rides a wave. Both techniques usually involve a supportive companion. Some women find that sitting in warm water reduces the pain of contractions. Others hire professional birth attendants called doulas. These women help the laboring woman as much as possible by massaging her, coaching her to breathe and push, and generally making her as comfortable as possible.

Epidurals

Most women who want anesthesia during labor get an epidural (see fig. 6). It is given by an anesthesiologist, who inserts a needle into a compartment around the woman's spinal cord. A thin plastic tube is threaded inside before withdrawing the needle. Painkiller is injected into the tube to keep the woman as comfortable as possible. This avoids the effects of giving systemic painkiller that enters the woman's blood-stream, then goes through the placenta into the baby. Women may get more painkiller as they need it if the initial dose starts to wear off.

Epidural medication has no contact with the baby's blood. It does not normally affect the baby at all, unless it lowers the mother's blood pressure and that goes unnoticed. It is important to get an epidural at the right time during active labor when it may help the woman relax and speed the opening of her cervix. An epidural that is given too early may interfere with the baby's normal descent and rotation, making labor longer than is necessary. Giving too much medicine, or giving it too late, may make it hard for the woman to push.

Even with an epidural, there are times when the woman will not be pain-free. The anesthesia may not completely mask the pain of the final

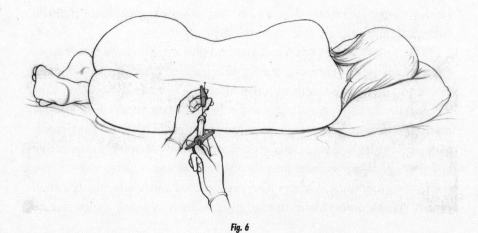

Fig. 6

stages of labor if that much medication will make it hard for the woman to push.

Epidurals given by a skilled anesthesiologist are very safe with only rare untoward consequences. Headaches are the most common side effect, occurring only 1 percent of the time. They are treated by giving a painkiller, or by injecting some of the patient's blood into the space from the epidural needle to patch the small hole. If left untreated, they usually go away within a week or two.

Although epidurals are often the pain medication of choice for labor, they cannot be given to some women. They include women whose blood doesn't clot properly (they have low platelet counts or are missing clotting factors), those with a Harrington rod (a rod that is surgically implanted into the back of a person with severe scoliosis), and those with fever (they may get an epidural abscess.) These women can get meperidine (Demerol), Stadol, or Nubain intravenously; they sedate both mother and baby.

The "twilight sleeps" that were common in our mothers' generations are rare today. Those were caused by giving large amounts of drugs like Demerol, together with a drug (scopolamine) that caused short-term memory loss. Today, pain control during labor and delivery should be worked out between a woman and her obstetrician, based on medical facts, not on anecdotal stories or false assumptions.

After Giving Birth

The third stage of labor is when the mother delivers the placenta. This can take anywhere from two to thirty minutes.

There is normally some brisk bleeding right after the placenta separates from the uterus. Most hospitals automatically give women Pitocin to cause uterine contractions to compress the blood vessels and slow the uterine bleeding. Some women have a uterus that does not contract well, and their large blood vessels stay open. This group includes women who have an overly distended uterus, those who had a very rapid or very long labor, those who received general anesthesia, and those who already gave birth to many children. When the uterus doesn't contract well, the caretaker vigorously massages the uterus and gives several medications that cause uterine contractions.

In those rare cases where the bleeding continues, radiologists can perform an almost miraculous procedure called arterial embolization. They thread small plastic catheters into the woman's groin and inject a substance into her bloodstream that clots off the major uterine arteries. This slows the blood flow to the uterus and lets the blood clot. This procedure is often life-saving, in addition to having spared many women the hysterectomy that must otherwise be done when all else fails.

Occasionally, heavy bleeding after delivery is due to a tear in the

246 · WHAT YOUR UNBORN BABY WANTS YOU TO KNOW

uterus, cervix, or vagina. That is remedied by stitching the wound. When it is due to a previously undiagnosed bleeding problem, the woman is given blood products that make up for what she is missing.

Once the uterine bleeding is controlled, the birth canal and cervix are examined for tears that need to be stitched. If an episiotomy was done, it is stitched now with dissolvable stitches that disappear during the next few days. The woman's legs are then lowered and she can sit up.

How do women feel after having a baby? After a first vaginal delivery with an episiotomy, they may feel pain for a week where they were cut. Walking during the first few days can be difficult. Initially applying ice packs to the perineum, followed by warm sitz baths several times a day, can reduce the swelling and discomfort.

With or without an episiotomy, first-time mothers usually feel very tired, especially if they breastfeed. Some women feel energized after subsequent deliveries, and need to make sure not to unduly stretch muscles or overexert themselves before their bodies return to normal. Of course, these are generalized reactions. Every individual and pregnancy is different.

After delivery, women have a vaginal discharge, called lochia, for several weeks to several months. It is bright red at first, with as much bleeding as a heavy period. It then becomes pinker and more mucous, then brown, then beige-yellow. If a woman exerts herself too much, the discharge may turn red again—she should take this as a warning to rest and relax for a bit.

Occasionally, a woman will start to bleed days or weeks after giving birth, usually because her uterus is not contracting properly. She should notify her caretaker if this happens. If it was not done right after delivery, the practitioner will make sure there are no fragments of placenta left inside her uterus, and treat a uterine infection if there is one.

Women should avoid sex as long as they bleed because they are more prone to getting pelvic infections then. After getting an episiotomy, sex is usually off-limits for the next six weeks.

CHAPTER TWENTY-FOUR

Being Overdue

O*nly 6 percent of babies are born on their due date. The overwhelm-*ing majority are born within a week of it. Six percent of babies are born "post-date." What does this mean, and what, if anything, should be done about it?

When a pregnant woman first sees her caretaker, the woman usually gets an approximate date when the baby is due to be born. This date is 280 days, or forty weeks, from the day her last menstrual period began. If a pregnancy lasts more than 294 days, or forty-two weeks, it is considered "postdate," and the baby is "overdue."

Due dates are not always accurate, especially when a woman does not know when her last period began or if her menstrual cycles vary in length. They are most accurate if a woman tested herself to see when she ovulated that month, or if she got pregnant using assisted fertility methods such as artificial insemination or IVF.

Another common, highly accurate way to set a due date is by measuring the embryo using ultrasound. By mid- or late pregnancy, a rough estimate of fetal age can also be made by measuring the height of the uterus (the fundus) in the woman's belly. The uterus is about the height of the woman's navel by midpregnancy. A week or two prior to delivery the height of the uterus usually drops a bit as the baby gets into position to be born, but this is not a definite predictor of impending labor. Women who are short- or long-waisted, or whose babies lie transversely, can have very different fundal heights.

Once a fairly accurate due date is known, it is easy to decide when a woman is postdate, or beyond the forty-second week of pregnancy.

Problems of Being Overdue

When a pregnancy goes beyond forty-two weeks, a baby is twice as likely as a full-term baby to have problems such as lack of oxygen, meconium, and even death. A baby born after forty-three weeks of pregnancy is three times as likely as a full-term baby to have these problems. This is because the placenta is likely to malfunction the longer the pregnancy continues.

In order to conceptualize this better, remember that the placenta is designed to work only a certain amount of time. When the pregnancy begins, the placenta normally works well and feeds the baby the way it should until forty weeks of pregnancy. After forty weeks the effectiveness of the placenta diminishes and can cause problems.

Shouldn't every baby, then, be delivered at the end of forty weeks? The answer is no. Inducing deliveries at the end of forty weeks would lead to an unnecessary number of cesarean sections. Also, if the cervix is not ripe or ready, inducing labor has some risks. Instead, the baby is watched carefully after forty-one weeks of gestation to make sure that the placenta is continually providing it with oxygen and nutrients. Beyond forty-two weeks, we believe the risk to the baby is too great so we routinely induce labor in any woman who goes beyond that point. Women with insulin-dependent diabetes, high blood pressure, or other risk factors may have their pregnancies interrupted earlier.

Monitoring Overdue Babies

We monitor overdue babies in several ways. The first is to tell the mother to perform a kick count every day, even though relying on the mother's perception of fetal activity is not enough by itself. A non-stress test can see if the baby is well oxygenated, and an ultrasound can see if there is enough amniotic fluid. If all three measures are normal, there is no reason to be concerned about a postdue baby. However, if any of these measures becomes abnormal, labor should be induced.

The moment the placenta starts malfunctioning there is a gradual decrease in amniotic fluid. This is because the placenta's primary job is to supply blood to the baby. If the baby does not get enough blood, it will not make a normal amount of urine. Since the amniotic fluid is made up of fetal urine, too little urine means too little amniotic fluid.

Thus, when the placenta malfunctions, the baby doesn't get enough blood and oxygen. It responds by feeding what it does get to its most vital organs—the heart and brain —and by depriving its kidneys. Since the kidneys have less blood to filter, less urine is made and excreted, and there is less amniotic fluid. This decrease in amniotic fluid can be seen quite easily on a fetal ultrasound.

Women often wonder why some babies are born normal after forty-two or forty-three weeks of pregnancy, while other postmature babies are not. We believe that some fetuses take longer than others to mature. Those babies who need more time do fine when they are born past their due dates. Those who don't need so much time look malnourished and old when they are born. Many of them have wrinkles, long nails, and dry skin.

The other problem that babies can have when they stay in the womb after they are mature is that they pass their first stool (meconium) there. That sometimes happens when they are deprived of oxygen. If they swallow meconium, they may have trouble breathing and may need special care for a long time.

Marianne was a twenty-three-year-old woman having her third baby. She had two previous normal, full-term deliveries but this time was one and a half weeks past her due date. Her obstetrician suggested inducing labor, but she was reluctant to have any unnecessary interventions. She then went to a high-risk specialist for a second opinion.

The specialist gave her a non-stress test, which was normal. He then measured her amniotic fluid using ultrasound, and it was also normal. She was advised to go home, rest, monitor her baby's movements using a kick count chart, and come back in three days for retesting. When Marianne came back, her non-stress test was still normal, but she no longer had enough amniotic fluid. The doctor felt strongly that the baby would not benefit from continuing the pregnancy and advised inducing labor. Marianne agreed. The baby was born with Apgar scores of 7 and 9, and was healthy. She is now three years old and is doing well.

CHAPTER TWENTY-FIVE

Cesarean Section

Today, *anywhere from 20 to 50 percent of babies in a given hospital* are delivered by cesarean section, with the national average in the United States being 25 percent. A cesarean section, or C-section, is the cutting open of the uterus in order to deliver a baby. When a baby will be delivered by cesarean section, a Foley catheter is placed in the mother's bladder to drain it and keep it empty. She then either gets more medication in an already-placed epidural or is given a spinal, epidural, or general anesthetic. A spinal and epidural are similar. A woman with either may feel pressure but no sharp pain, and some short-lived nausea when the doctor manipulates the tissue in the abdomen.

General anesthesia is only used when very necessary, such as when there is sudden fetal distress or the woman has a bleeding abnormality, a high fever, hemorrhage, or a significant back deformity.

A screen will be placed on the woman that prevents her from viewing the cesarean. The doctor makes a six-inch sideways cut through the skin just above the pubic bone. The layers of tissue underneath are then cut through until the abdominal cavity can be opened and all of its organs can be seen. The bladder is moved down and the uterus is cut open. The baby is removed immediately and its umbilical cord is cut. Since the cut uterus bleeds a lot, it is sewn back together as quickly as possible.

The other layers of tissue are then sewn up, and the skin is closed with staples, silk stitches that will need to be removed, or invisible dissolving stitches.

A cesarean section usually takes anywhere from thirty to ninety minutes. When the fetus is distressed, the baby is normally delivered in less than two minutes from the time the incision is made! Having had a prior cesarean section, or being obese, makes the surgery harder.

Women have pain during the twenty-four to forty-eight hours after a cesarean section, which necessitates pain pumps, shots, or pills like Percocet. They needn't worry about the drugs getting into their breast milk because they make mostly colostrum at this time. Most women feel much better by the third or fourth day. Around the fourth day, staples and removable stitches are taken out.

Women who have had cesarean sections normally feel weaker and less energetic than other new mothers. The abdominal surgery sometimes necessitates taking painkillers for a week or two. The incision site is usually sore and red, with the skin on top being numb, while nearby skin is raised and hard. It may take as long as a year to go back to normal.

Women who had C-sections have a postpartum bloody discharge as they shed their uterine lining, just as happens after a vaginal delivery. Women can start exercising six weeks later, but they should start slowly and gradually increase the length and difficulty of their sessions.

Why Cesarean Sections Are Done

There are many reasons that doctors do cesarean sections. Some reasons include:

1. There was a prior cesarean section. Many cesarean sections in the past were done simply because there was a prior C-section. Nowadays, women who had a prior cesarean section are usually encouraged to try vaginal delivery (VBAC—vaginal birth after cesarean).

2. Labor doesn't progress, or the baby can't fit through the pelvis. Many babies are too big to fit through their mother's pelvis. At other times, the uterine contractions are not effective at pushing the baby out.

Some babies are positioned such that they can't emerge vaginally. Any of these three situations may result in a cesarean section.

3. There is fetal distress. When a fetus isn't getting enough oxygen, or is too distressed by labor, a cesarean section will get the baby out quickly.

4. The baby is breech. Most obstetricians prefer to deliver breech babies by cesarean section rather than vaginally.

5. There is a multiple gestation. Almost all triplets and higher order multiples are delivered by C-section, as are many twins.

6. The baby is severely premature. Very premature babies have less stamina than full-term ones, and they often can't tolerate labor. They also tend to be breech or transverse more than others. These babies are usually delivered by cesarean section.

7. The mother has placenta previa. When the woman's placenta covers the cervix, a cesarean section is the only way to deliver the baby.

8. There has been a placental abruption. When the placenta detaches from the uterine wall, a cesarean section is done unless vaginal delivery is imminent.

9. The umbilical cord has prolapsed. The baby's blood supply is cut off when the cord drops through the open cervix, ahead of the baby. Doing a cesarean section is usually the only way to get the baby out quickly enough.

10. The baby is known to be very big. A large baby can make vaginal delivery very difficult, especially if it is a woman's first birth.

11. The mother has genital herpes. A woman must deliver by cesarean section if she has active genital herpes.

Increase in Cesarean Sections

Many reasons are given for why cesarean sections are done so much more often today than a generation or two ago:

1. Many more cesarean sections are being done, so more women are having repeat C-sections.

2. American women are delaying childbearing. Women who have their first child later in life need forceps or cesarean sections more often than younger women. Older mothers have more complications such as diabetes and high blood pressure that make C-sections more likely. They may also have more rigid pelvises, less effective pushing, and more fetal distress due to placenta problems.

3. Most breech babies are delivered by cesarean section today. While most vaginally delivered breech babies do well, there is a small chance that a breech's arm will get stuck behind the head, or the head will get stuck in the mother's pelvis.

4. Obstetricians are petrified by the ever-looming threat of lawsuits, and they are sued more than any other doctors. Consequently, many doctors will choose C-section and err on the side of caution.

5. Forceps and vacuum are used less often. Women often don't like these ways of assisting delivery. When a woman can't push the baby out the last little bit, or if there is sudden fetal distress and the baby's head is not quite out, a cesarean section must be done if forceps or vacuum are ruled out.

6. More women than ever are conceiving through assisted fertility techniques, which often result in multiple pregnancies. As we mentioned earlier, multiple pregnancies often have risks that result in at least one baby being delivered by cesarean section.

7. More American women are obese today. Obese women are more likely to require a C-section and are more likely than normal-weight women to produce big babies.

Vaginal Birth after Cesarean Section (VBAC)

Cesarean sections were once done by cutting the thick layers of the uterus from top to bottom, which weakens the uterus a lot. Since scar tissue doesn't stretch as well as muscle, the pregnant uterus will tend to rip along its scar, with potentially catastrophic results. This is because the huge blood vessels that feed the pregnant uterus will lead to a hemorrhage if they rip. When that happens, the baby must be delivered immediately, and extensive surgery with transfusions for the mother are needed.

When doctors started cutting the uterus horizontally near the cervix where the uterine wall is thinner, the scars ruptured less often during subsequent pregnancies. When VBACs are successful, as they usually are, recovery is quicker, and the delivery is usually as easy as with women who have never had a C-section. This is a great advantage since cesarean sections inherently have a greater risk of complications than vaginal deliveries.

While vaginal birth after this type of cesarean section is often safe, the uterus may still rupture up to 1 percent of the time. It seems that many of the uterine ruptures after cesarean section happened when labor was induced. This is why some obstetricians prefer not to induce such women. Still, each labor has its own circumstances. Sometimes it seems clear that the labor will be successful, while other times it is obvious that labor will not be productive and a cesarean section will be needed. A recent study suggests that the safety of a VBAC is maximized when 18 months elapse between the C-section and the next pregnancy.

Women who attempt VBAC should have their labor continuously monitored, as fetal distress may be the first sign that the uterus has ruptured. If women are anesthetized, they can't feel the terrible pain of the uterus tearing.

Cesarean sections can be life-saving under certain circumstances, and be done to avoid potential problems in others. Like any surgical procedure, the decision to do a C-section may be a complex one with a mixture of pros and cons.

PART IV

Postpartum

CHAPTER TWENTY-SIX

The Newborn Baby

No book on pregnancy could be complete without discussing the long-awaited, eagerly anticipated baby. Despite the many months of waiting for this tiny guest of honor to join them, parents must now make a drastic shift from expectant to actual parents. This is totally different from any other role they have played before. Juggling the different needs of multiple family members with those of a new baby can be daunting even for a super-mom. It can be overwhelming, and even terrifying, for a first-time mother. We hope this chapter will help new mothers get started, but please also read articles and books about what to expect during the first year of a baby's life.

When the baby emerges from the mother's body, the mother may expect to see a small, pink, round face and head and perfectly formed, pudgy body. Instead, newborns are covered with a slimy red and white mixture of the mother's blood, amniotic fluid, and often vernix. (The vernix is the creamy lotion that keeps babies from turning into prunes after a nine-month-long bath.)

Instead of having a perfectly round head, the baby is more likely to look like a conehead with a misshapen and lopsided head. This is because the skull bones get squished when the baby's head moves through the birth canal, and it takes a day or two for the bones to separate and return to their proper places. This is why babies have fontanels, or "soft spots" on the tops and backs of their heads. Without them, the baby could not get its head through the mother's vagina. As the baby gets older, the skull bones grow and fuse together.

Occasionally a newborn has large blood clots, or hematomas, on the head. These are not dangerous but take a few days to disappear. A third or more of newborns have deep pink splotches on their skin, usually on the forehead, upper eyelids, or back of the neck. These discolorations, or "stork marks," are many superficial blood vessels that fade away during the first few years. Many babies have an insignificant little rash made up of clusters of little white bumps called "milia."

Babies born by cesarean section usually look "better" than those born vaginally because their heads do not get compressed during the birth process. While the baby's face and torso should be pink or ruddy, his hands and feet are usually bluish. Fetuses get less oxygen through the umbilical cord, and it takes awhile for the newly oxygenated lungs to pump well-oxygenated blood to the baby's hands and feet.

After delivery, the baby's mouth and nose are suctioned out carefully with a long, flexible tube. This not only removes mucus and secretions, but hopefully removes any meconium before the baby breathes it in and forces it into his lungs.

The umbilical cord hangs from the baby's belly until it is cut and clamped. Some practitioners then dry off the baby, wrap him in a soft towel or blanket, and give him to the mother to hold or put to the breast. It is important that the baby not get chilled. He is used to being in a tropical environment that is a constant 98.6 degrees, and the delivery room is much colder than that. Since a third of the body's heat is lost through our heads, newborns get caps to help them keep warm.

Some practitioners put babies under a warmer as soon as the umbilical cord is cut, while the pediatrician or nurse takes a look. If the baby's head and torso are pink, that is a good sign. If they are very pale or blue, a caretaker will help the baby breathe better. Mottled skin is a sign that the baby is cold or has an infection. Very red skin means the baby got too much blood when his mother's blood suddenly spilled into his, or from a twin's blood supply.

When the baby's body and lips are pink but the face is deep blue, it is usually from broken facial blood vessels. This happens when an umbilical cord is tightly wrapped around the baby's neck, when there was a difficult delivery of the shoulders, or when the baby's head sat on the mother's perineum for a while. It is nothing to worry about. The blue color will fade over a couple of days.

The doctor notes the baby's heart and breathing rates and muscle tone. A normal newborn averages 160 heartbeats per minute, with a range of 120–200, and breathes sixty times a minute during the first hour. A newborn should cry vigorously; a feeble or high-pitched cry warrants attention. The baby is weighed and measured either in the delivery room or in the nursery.

Hospitals routinely give vitamin K injections to all newborns because some babies don't have a clotting factor and vitamin K helps blood clot. The nurse puts silver nitrate drops or erythromycin ointment into newborns' eyes. This is because babies whose mothers have chlamydia or gonorrhea (both sexually transmitted diseases) can get a form of conjunctivitis that may damage the eyes if it is not treated. Rather than treat only the very small number of babies who need vitamin K or eye antibiotics, many states mandate that all babies get them.

If the baby seems healthy, he gets an identification bracelet put on his ankle and his footprint is taken. Then, he is given to the mother to bond and/or nurse. If the baby has problems, he may be taken to the nursery. Mothers find it very distressing to have such longed-for babies spirited away almost as soon as they arrive, but babies are only removed if they are deemed to need medical intervention.

Even if the baby is healthy, he is soon taken away to the nursery, unless the mother is in a hospital that allows the baby to stay with her. In either case, he will be watched closely during the first few hours. Most nurseries will bathe the baby, which often chills him and necessitates rewarming him under a warmer. If a mother doesn't want the baby to be bathed, or wants only the head and face bathed, she can request that. If the baby is very big or very small, he may get his blood glucose checked.

Newborns are likely to show signs of trouble during the first few hours if they have an infection or immature lungs or a significant defect like a heart problem that wasn't noticed at birth. Even when the baby stays in the mother's room, hospital staff will be keeping a close watch on her baby.

Some women are concerned that someone at the hospital will mix up their baby with someone else's. Hospitals are very vigilant about this now. They immediately put a wrist band with the mother's name on the mother as soon as she is admitted, and the baby gets an identical name band on the ankle as soon as it is born. These bands can only be removed by cutting them. Some hospitals even use alarmed tags like those used to tag clothing in stores. The tags set off alarms if the babies are brought past certain doors.

The mother should not leave her baby alone to go to the bathroom or to take a shower. Most hospital abductions occur when women leave the infant alone to use the bathroom. Ask a nurse to watch the baby or bring it back to the nursery until you are ready to take it.

Circumcision

Circumcision is the cutting off of the foreskin of the penis. Jewish ritual circumcision, known as a bris, is performed by a mohel (an expert in performing circumcisions) when a boy is eight days old. This religious ceremony is usually attended by the baby's parents, family, and friends. Muslims also circumcise their sons for religious reasons.

Many American babies that will not have a circumcision for ritual reasons will be circumcised in the hospital, but this is not done in most of the rest of the world.

While the religious basis for ritual circumcision is wholly spiritual, and has nothing to do with hygiene, the rationale for circumcising boys in hospitals is that smegma and dirt can accumulate under the foreskin if it is not cleaned well. Also, uncircumcised men may have a greater incidence of penile cancer. Some studies have suggested that women who have sex with uncircumcised men may have a greater chance of infections as well.

A social consideration for many American parents is that they want their boys to look like their peers. Because circumcision is the norm, they don't want their sons to look different from his friends or from his father. At the present time, some people are questioning the rationale for circumcising babies for nonritual reasons. Recent studies show that circumcised boys have fewer urinary infections than other boys do. Parents who are undecided about whether or not to circumcise their boys for nonritual reasons should discuss the pros and cons with their pediatrician.

Jaundice

Jaundice in newborns results from the inability of the baby's liver to get rid of broken-down red blood cells fast enough. This makes the baby look yellow. While many premature babies have some jaundice, and a smaller percentage of full-term babies also do, it is potentially dangerous to the baby. A mother may be ready to take her baby home on the second day after delivery, but the pediatrician may inform her that the baby needs to stay under strong lights in the incubator to get rid of jaundice. Most of the time, jaundice is nothing worrisome and it goes away within two or three days. The bright lights help the chemicals that cause the jaundice break down and be excreted more quickly.

Sometimes babies go home and the mothers notice that the baby becomes more orangey or yellow during the first week. If you press your finger into the baby's skin, then take your finger away, the baby's skin should not look as yellow as a lemon. If it does, speak to your pediatrician.

Breastfeeding can temporarily exacerbate jaundice, but that is no reason to stop nursing. Keeping a mildly jaundiced baby in daylight (making sure that it is not exposed to direct sunlight, where it could get burned) is a good way to reduce the jaundice.

Diapering

Babies are best diapered with as few chemicals as possible. Avoid using baby wipes when wet cotton balls or a moist, soft cotton cloth will do. If the baby's bottom is irritated, try using Balmex, Desitin, calendula cream, or unpetroleum jelly (the latter two are available in health food stores). A baby's stools can break down its delicate skin, so dirty diapers should be changed as soon as possible.

New parents are often concerned that a baby's stools look different from an adult's, especially if the baby is breastfed. They will be the color of mustard, watery, frequent, and will not smell very bad. Once a baby starts eating foods besides breast milk, dirty diapers will smell characteristically like dirty diapers.

It should be noted that some breastfed babies will have wet diapers frequently, but after the first few months may not have a bowel movement for days or weeks at a time. Some babies at three months or older even go for two weeks at a time before they have a bowel movement. If they don't appear uncomfortable, nothing needs to be done about it. In such cases the breast milk is so well digested and absorbed that there is not enough waste to make the baby move his bowels very often.

Burping

Babies must be burped after each feeding because they suck in air which can otherwise get trapped in their stomachs and cause painful gas. Babies can be burped by holding them upright after a feeding, chin over the parent's shoulder, and gently patting their back until you hear the rewarding rush of gas from their mouth. Occasionally, babies who are breastfed do not need to be burped after every feeding, and some don't need to be burped at all. If you spend five or more minutes trying unsuccessfully to get the baby to burp, don't go crazy. Your baby may not need to burp. If this happens repeatedly, and the baby does not seem to be uncomfortable, you may not need to burp your baby unless it seems distressed.

Spitting Up

Every baby digests food differently, and they are not born knowing when they are full, or how much food they need to eat. Some babies rarely spit up, while others can soak through several changes of theirs and their mother's clothes every morning.

Vomiting is different than spitting up. Spitting up occurs when babies gently regurgitate one to several mouthfuls of food soon after eating. Vomiting is forceful. In projectile vomiting the baby's muscles send the stomach contents flying across the room, sometimes as much as several feet away. This can happen when the baby is allergic to food or formula or when there is a gastrointestinal problem that needs medical attention. When projectile vomiting occurs, the pediatrician should be contacted.

Colic

Colic is a mysterious form of abdominal pain of unknown cause. It usually starts when babies are between two and four weeks old, and usually ends magically at three months, although it can occasionally go into the fourth month. Every day, the baby gets fussier and fussier, starting in the late afternoon or early evening. Soon, the baby is screaming in pain, with his legs tucked up into his abdomen and his fists clenched tightly. He seems to be looking for food, but will pull his face away if the breast or bottle is offered. He is very gassy, indicating that the pain is coming from the abdomen. These hours of screaming are extraordinarily trying for even seasoned parents because little seems to help.

Some babies calm down with rocking, or being held while the parent walks incessantly throughout the house. Some babies may stop screaming only if they are held upright, or in a certain position in a baby carrier, or tummy-down on a parent's legs while their back is stroked. When the pain is bad, some babies calm down when they are held (carefully) in a warm bath. Others do well when they are held while sucking on an empty breast or a pacifier. Some parents even swear that turning on the vacuum cleaner soothes their colicky infants.

Colicky babies should be kept nearly upright during feedings, and burping should never be neglected. Babies can be offered some warm (not hot) chamomile tea, or Mylicon Drops to help soothe away the gas.

Parents of colicky babies will find that everyone is an expert on how to calm down their child. Unfortunately, more often than not having a colicky baby is a torturous experience that seems to have no end. One parent of a colicky adopted child expressed, in a moment of honesty, what many parents feel, "If my wife didn't love this baby so much, we would have thrown it out the window a long time ago."

Parents need to know that colic is common, the baby and they will be fine, and the problem will go away on its own in a few months. Until that happens, parents need to be reassured that parenthood after the colic stops can really be the wonderful experience it is.

ﾐ CHAPTER TWENTY-SEVEN

Postpartum Blues

Postpartum blues, those periods of sadness and loneliness in the weeks after having a baby, occur in 50 percent of women. They are so common that they are almost considered normal for new mothers. Apart from the sleep deprivation that occurs with a new baby, the physical discomfort in the genital area or breasts coupled with hormonal swings as the body readjusts can be daunting. Pregnancy, despite its discomforts, had a certain magic, with the wonderful anticipation of a baby who stretched and kicked and curled up inside. Now, the reality may be very different than that idealized fantasy, and any problem that arises may magnify that disappointment. The baby is suddenly physically separate from the mother and very, very needy. The mother has no privacy, and no time to call her own. If the baby is colicky or there is a stressful marriage, demanding children, or inadequate support, chances are good that a woman will experience those famous blues.

Giving birth can also reawaken past traumas, such as giving birth to a stillborn child, repeated miscarriages, or the heartbreak during stressful years of fruitless infertility treatments. One might think that a previously infertile woman who has now achieved the goal of her efforts would be delighted. In fact, many such women find themselves reliving the pain of their past.

If a woman accepts her painful feelings as being normal, and allows herself to grieve and cry out her pent-up emotions, they will usually pass within a few weeks. Most women get through their adjustment period within a month with little more than a feeling of upset and occasional crying.

On the other hand, postpartum depression is indistinguishable from other forms of depression, except that childbirth triggers it. The life changes that a new baby brings may be traumatic. Women may grieve over irreparably losing their freedom or giving up their jobs. They may reexperience the pain of lacking their own mothering when they were growing up. They may feel inadequate in their ability to mother their new baby, and have a profound lack of self-esteem.

Postpartum depression is characterized by a pervasive feeling of sadness and not being able to enjoy anything. The person cannot be cheered up. She feels as if a dark cloud is hanging over her that never goes away, and a heavy weight rests on her shoulders. Her lethargy makes everything seem like an unbearable burden. She will usually have difficulty sleeping, although occasionally a woman will sleep so much that she rarely gets out of bed. She may neglect the baby, about whom she may seem to be almost frighteningly detached. She dislikes herself, and may even reach a point of seeing no reason to live. On occasion, a woman might feel suicidal, and even want to kill her baby with her.

Women with postpartum depression need professional help as soon as possible. That may include psychotherapy, sometimes medication, and, rarely, hospitalization. Many women feel better after a few weeks, although for some it will take longer. Most women do recover from postpartum depression, although it tends to recur after subsequent births. For this reason, some doctors start their patients on antidepressants a few days after delivering. Being prepared and getting support systems in place before giving birth tends to help a lot.

CHAPTER TWENTY-EIGHT

Breastfeeding

The best and most easily provided nourishment for the baby is that which the mother produces herself. Unfortunately, new mothers and new babies often have a frustrating period of adjustment starting right after the baby is born. While some babies will nurse hungrily when put to the breast after delivery, others are so exhausted from their stressful journey that they would much rather sleep! Babies may not want to wake up for feedings during the intervals when the hospital staff is scheduled to bring the newborn to the mother. Newborns sometimes have a hard time latching onto the breast. They also take a long time to learn when their tummies are too full, and they commonly spit up their feedings. Babies are not used to this new way of eating because they didn't have to do this in the uterus.

It is unfortunate that many hospitals only bring newborns to their mothers every four hours for thirty to forty-five minutes. This makes it difficult for many mothers to nurse when the baby is hungry and awake. Breastfeeding mothers should nurse their babies "on demand," meaning when the baby indicates that he is hungry. Nursing infants often need to nurse every two and a half to three hours, and some hospitals give the babies sugar water or formula in the nursery if the babies are hungry between scheduled feedings. This further interferes with the mother's ability to nurse because the baby is asleep and not hungry when it is brought to her.

How does one breastfeed a newborn? The mother first strokes her baby's cheek. It will turn its head, or root, in the direction of her finger. Then the mother puts her nipple and as much of the areola (the dark area around the nipple) as will comfortably fit into the baby's mouth. Since most of the milk ducts are under the areola, the more areola in the baby's mouth, the more milk he can get. The mother may need to make a space for the baby to breathe by pressing her thumb against her breast so that it doesn't cover the baby's nose. Since all new babies breathe through their noses, the baby will not be able to breathe if the mother's skin blocks the way.

During the first twenty-four to forty-eight hours of the baby's life, the mother and baby need to learn how to latch on so that the mother's nipples don't become very sore. If the nipples crack or bleed, the pain of the baby's mouth when nursing will spoil the experience for the mother. If needed, women can apply a breast cream containing lanolin, aloe, and/or vitamin E. It is available without a prescription at pharmacies or at health food stores. It soothes, moisturizes, and heals sore nipples.

A major reason that breastfeeding fails is that mothers get bad advice. Many hospitals have lactation specialists who teach new mothers how to breastfeed and overcome problems that arise. If your hospital doesn't have one, ask your practitioner to recommend someone before the baby arrives. Making a connection with this specialist before the need arises can nip many problems in the bud.

Colostrum and Milk Supply

When the baby is born, the mother's breasts produce a rich, yellow secretion called colostrum. It is chock-full of nutrients and antibodies that help the baby fight infections. On the second or third day after delivery, the mother's milk arrives, engorging her breasts and making them feel sore. If she feeds the baby as he gets hungry, her breasts will soon feel better.

The nursing mother's and baby's bodies have an exquisite interdependence. The more milk the baby needs, the more he nurses, and the more the mother's breasts are stimulated to supply. The size of a woman's breasts have nothing to do with how well they provide. The amount of stimulation they get from the baby sucking primarily determines how much milk is produced.

If a woman is bottle-feeding, her breasts will be sore for a few days after her milk comes in. Women no longer get injections to stop them from making milk. They simply wear a good bra, don't empty the breasts or stimulate their nipples, and apply ice packs as needed.

It is normal for a breastfed baby to lose as much as a half pound between the time of delivery and the time he leaves the hospital. Don't worry—he'll gain the weight back soon enough. Mothers often worry since they can't gauge how much breast milk the baby is getting, it might not be enough. Newborns should wet a diaper during their first twenty-four hours and have a bowel movement within the first forty-eight. After that, a baby should wet six to eight diapers a day. If he's doing this, he's getting plenty of milk from the mother. Bear in mind that today's disposable diapers are so absorbent that babies may urinate much more frequently than is evident by looking at, or even touching, the diaper. If the baby is weighed during the first few weeks after birth, it will be obvious if the baby is gaining weight or not. If you have concerns, don't start supplementing with formula. Speak to a lactation specialist and/or your pediatrician for support and reassurance.

It is perfectly normal for breastfed babies to gain less weight than their bottle-fed neighbors, and to feed more often. Bottle-fed babies have a greater risk of obesity, so bigger is not necessarily better. The fact that a breastfed baby needs to nurse every hour and a half to two hours does not mean that the mother isn't making enough milk. Breast milk is much more digestible than bottled milk, so it leaves the stomach more rapidly and the baby consequently needs to nurse more often.

When we speak about how often a baby nurses, the time between feedings is counted from the time the baby first starts to the next time the baby starts. If a newborn takes thirty minutes to nurse, it may well start feeding again an hour and a half or two hours after it stops. If someone asks you how often that baby is nursing, the answer is every two to two and a half hours.

It is easy to see why nursing mothers can be so exhausted when they nurse eight to twelve times around the clock for as much as thirty or forty minutes at a time. Bottle-fed babies can drink their formula faster than most infants can nurse, and bottle-fed babies can often go longer between feedings. This should not deter new mothers from having the patience to give their babies the perfect baby food. Not only is breast milk far superior to formula in ways too numerous to mention, but after a short while breastfeeding will also be much more convenient than bottle-feeding. There are no solutions to mix, no cans to open, no bottles to sterilize, no need to warm up the milk, no need to haul around bottles and the like. The woman need only open her shirt and dinner is warm, waiting, nourishing and delicious, wherever the baby and mother are.

Don't give a bottle of formula to a breastfed baby to see if the baby is hungry or not. If the baby is hungry, putting him on the breast as often as is necessary will soon result in the mother making more milk. Diverting that stimulation to a bottle whenever the baby seems "too hungry" will result in the mother's milk supply dwindling more and more.

If the pediatrician tells the mother that the baby is indeed not gaining enough weight, the mother might need to improve her diet, drink more fluids, and get more rest. Fatigue, missing meals, and lack of nutritious food can play havoc with some women's milk production. Those who favor alternative remedies may find that taking a daily vitamin B-complex with 25 milligrams each of B_1, B_2, and B_6 helps, as do teas made from herbs such as fennel seed, anise, and licorice. These herbs have a long history of being used to stimulate milk production. Formulations containing herbs, such as Mother's Milk, a tea made by Traditional Medicinals, are available in most health food stores.

If you still aren't making enough milk and need to supplement, consult a lactation specialist. She can show you how to use a syringe and thin plastic tube to feed the baby and stimulate your milk supply at the same time, besides offering other suggestions.

Mastitis

Breastfeeding is not always as easy as it looks. Some women get plugged milk ducts that cause an area of the breast to become hard and very sore. It will usually go back to normal in two to three days, which can seem like an eternity, if the woman does the following: She should massage the hard area by repeatedly pressing down in the direction of the nipple to try to force the milk out. She can run hot water over it in the shower or put hot, wet towels or a hot pack on it, making sure not to burn the sensitive breast skin. She should also make sure to empty the breast as often as possible by feeding the baby or pumping her milk.

In mastitis, the breast is red, hot, and very sore. The woman feels sick, and she can get a high fever. The woman needs to do the same things that she does for a plugged duct, but she will also need antibiotics if she has an infection. She can usually keep breastfeeding because the mastitis is caused by bacteria that came from the baby's mouth! Mastitis usually resolves without causing further problems. Rarely, additional medical attention is necessary.

Nursing Clothes

New breastfeeding mothers discover a lot by trial and error. Right away they find out that many of their prepregnancy clothes are completely unsuitable because they are closed in front. Nursing shirts, dresses, and even nightgowns and pajamas have inconspicuous flaps in front that let women nurse discreetly almost anywhere. They can be bought from catalogs or in most maternity stores.

Some breastfeeding women find that their breasts leak milk at times. This can happen when the breasts are full of milk, or when thoughts of their baby stimulate the "let-down" reflex, and milk squirts out. (This can also happen during sex.) Women for whom this is a problem can buy cotton pads called breast shields that are placed inside the bra and changed as needed. These are available in pharmacies and maternity stores.

Now that they have given birth, some women are very anxious to return to their prepregnancy weight. Well-meaning women will tell new mothers, "The weight will just melt off of you once you start nursing." Other equally well-meaning women will insist, "You'll never be able to lose weight while you're nursing." Both are true for different women. Since nursing mothers need to get about five hundred calories a day more than when not nursing, some women will not make up the caloric demands and will lose weight rapidly. Others will find they are exhausted, sedentary, and have a voracious appetite. They not only don't lose weight, they gain.

Strict dieting is not a good idea, as it can reduce the milk supply, but eating a bit less than is needed to maintain your weight will lead to gradual weight loss. Moderate exercise will not only help you lose the extra pregnancy weight, it will help tone your body. During the first six postpartum weeks be sure to avoid exercises that strain or stretch the abdomen or perineal region. It is best to feed the baby before strenuous exercise because the exercise can make the milk taste unappealing. Once a baby is a few months old, she can drink a quart of milk a day. Make sure to drink lots of fluids before and after any exercise to replenish what you lose.

How long should a mother breastfeed? Whatever she can do is great. At least six to twelve months is ideal, and many mothers continue until their children are two or even three years old. Having an encouraging and supportive husband and pediatrician can make an enormous difference in the choice a woman makes about how long to nurse.

Breast Pumps

Going back to work need not interfere with a woman's decision to breastfeed. She can breastfeed her baby while she is at home, and pump her milk while at work. Some women do this for as long as two years.

Two basic kinds of pumps are available. Manual pumps require a woman to squeeze a handle repeatedly so that a suction is created by a plastic "hood" over her nipple. As the milk is drawn out, it flows into a baby bottle below. Electric or battery-operated pumps do the woman's work for her. Manual pumps are usually purchased, while the more expensive electric ones are either purchased or rented. A woman can also express milk by rolling her nipples between her thumb and forefinger, but this is too time-consuming for most busy women today.

To pump milk at work, all that is needed is a private room, a good pump, and an electric socket if an electric pump is being used. The woman should wear clothing that opens easily in front and will not be stained if some milk leaks or spills.

If a nursing woman needs to travel, some battery-operated pumps even have adaptors that can be plugged into the cigarette lighter of a car! Traveling by plane can be more difficult. Make sure to bring a non-electric pump if you might need to pump in an airplane bathroom. Almost no airplanes have live electric sockets anymore, even though the outlets are there. They have almost universally been deactivated. Also, airport bathrooms do not have working electric sockets in the stalls. No one wants to pump milk in front of public sinks! In an emergency, an airline executive club might have a private room they will let you use.

Expressed or pumped milk will keep two days in the refrigerator and at least two weeks in the freezer. Ice packs used in small coolers can keep the milk cold if no refrigerator is available until you get home.

Some women will choose not to, or won't be able to, breastfeed. They should not be made to feel guilty. While breast milk is the ideal, formula has been used to nourish babies for decades. Whether women breastfeed or not, their most important role as mothers remains.

CHAPTER TWENTY-NINE

The Postpartum Visit

*W*omen *normally see their practitioner six weeks after giving birth. It* takes this long for the body to go back to its normal state whether delivery was vaginal or by cesarean section. The practitioner will check the woman's blood pressure to make sure that she does not have on-going hypertension and to make sure that episiotomy or cesarean section scars are healing properly. This is also a good time to examine a woman's breasts, although it may be hard to do this if a woman is breast-feeding.

Resuming Sex

Typically, the most pressing questions women have during this visit are about when they can resume sex, and what they can do to prevent pregnancy so soon after delivery. Unless there are complications such as infection or unhealed scars or tears, doctors generally consider it safe for women to resume having sex by six weeks after childbirth. Around the time of this postpartum visit, most women will resume having sex, although women differ widely in this regard. Women in some parts of the world do not have sex at all until they stop breastfeeding. On the other hand, over 90 percent of the women in western Europe, North America, Australia, Japan, and other industrialized countries resume having sex six weeks after giving birth. Breastfeeding women in America tend to resume having sex a week or two later than women who don't breastfeed.

Many women will find they need to use lubricant for a while in order for intercourse to feel comfortable, especially if they are breastfeeding. The hormones that facilitate nursing keep estrogen levels low, and this may make the vagina uncomfortably dry, at least during the first few months. Doing Kegel exercises may help improve vaginal tone.

These issues aside, the biggest obstacle to sex for most new mothers is their overwhelming fatigue. Exhaustion depresses libido, and the opportunity to sleep often seems more appealing than sex. While an average couple may have sex twice a week or more before having children, the average frequency of sex after having children is about once a week.

Until some women lose most of their pregnancy weight, or their muscles return to normal, they may feel less than sexy. Listening for the newborn's cries during lovemaking also dampens one's ardor. Obviously, women who suffer from postpartum blues will be uninterested in sex, among many other things.

What can a couple do to improve their sex life after having a baby? First, try to get enough help for the new mother that she is not constantly exhausted, whether this means accepting help from friends and family or hiring help. Two, consider making love at times of opportunity, not necessarily at night. Early in the morning or during a baby's afternoon nap can be excellent times for intimacy. Taking a shower or bath together, cuddling in bed, and physical contact without having intercourse don't have to fall by the wayside.

Three, some women need a lot of reassurance that they are still attractive to their husbands, even when their bodies are not what they used to be. By the same token, many men need to feel they are still desirable when a woman seems so focused on the new baby, and often prefers sleeping to being with them. A man shouldn't take it personally when his wife doesn't have the same sexual interest in him that she had before having a baby. Changes in hormone levels, exhaustion, and many new stresses are probably to blame.

If a couple finds that more than three months have passed without having sex and this is upsetting one or both partners, or that five months after having a baby their sex life is still not satisfying, marriage counseling might be helpful.

Contraception

Practitioners usually discuss birth control with their patients during the postpartum visit. This is because women who do not breastfeed generally start to ovulate about forty-five days after giving birth, although some women ovulate as soon as twenty-five days after delivery.

Ninety-eight percent of women who breastfeed exclusively and frequently, and who do not get a period, will have natural contraception for the first six months after giving birth. Women who want nursing to double as a contraception should make sure not to let more than four hours go by without nursing during the day, or more than six hours at night. If a woman uses a pump instead of nursing, the contraceptive effect of nursing is not as dependable because the baby sucks more vigorously than the pump mimics.

Coitus interruptus, or withdrawing the penis from the vagina before ejaculating, is one of the oldest forms of birth control and is used widely throughout the world. It is not completely reliable for several reasons. First, there may be sperm in the penile fluid that wets the penis long before ejaculation occurs.

A second reason why coitus interruptus is not recommended for birth control is that the ejaculate may end up around the vulva, where the sperm can travel up the vagina into the uterus and fallopian tube. A final reason is that the man may have the best of intentions but still not withdraw in time.

The rhythm method is also unreliable because a woman may either have irregular periods or have one irregular cycle. In addition, a woman's libido is often highest around the time of ovulation, when conception is most likely to occur, and lowest at "safe" times. Finally, sperm that are in the woman's body can live for days. Conception has been reported when ovulation occurred as long as a week later.

A diaphragm is a round latex device that looks like a small frisbee. It is put deep into the vagina so that it covers the cervix. The woman must coat it on the outside and fill it on the inside with spermicidal jelly every time before having sex. Thus, the cervix sits in a pool of spermicide. It must be left in place for at least six hours after intercourse.

Women must be fitted with a diaphragm by a practitioner, and refitted every time a woman gains or loses twenty pounds. It must also be replaced every two years. Some women can't use it because their fingers can't place it properly; others develop urinary tract infections when they use diaphragms. The failure rate of diaphragms also goes up with the number of babies a woman has.

Spermicide can be obtained as cream, jelly, aerosol, tablet, suppository, or film (VCF). It is often used alone, especially when contraception is needed for only a short time. It is usually less effective than using a diaphragm, so using a double application is recommended. When conception occurs after using spermicide, it does not cause birth defects.

Condoms are sheaths made of latex or animal intestine. They are put on an erect penis before intercourse so that there is some empty space hanging at the end. This allows semen to be ejaculated inside it. If the penis is not withdrawn before it becomes completely soft afterward, a condom may fall off and spill some of its contents into the vagina. Condoms also break on occasion.

Condoms are considered to be the most effective barrier method of contraception, and those with spermicide on them are best. Condoms can also protect against venereal diseases and HIV. Latex condoms are better than natural ones for this purpose.

Female condoms, polyurethane pouches that go over the vulva and extend into the vagina, were developed as a way of preventing the spread of venereal diseases. They are not used much.

There are two kinds of intrauterine devices (IUDs), which, when put in the uterus, interfere with sperm traveling through the uterus to the fallopian tube. IUDs also change the uterine lining so that it is hard for fertilized eggs to implant there. It was originally thought that IUDs worked by causing mini-abortions, but it is now known that they primarily prevent fertilization.

The Paraguard is used almost exclusively. It is made of copper and needs to be replaced every ten years. Progestasert has hormones in it and needs to be replaced every year.

IUDs may increase menstrual pain and flow. It is a good form of birth control, but the rare complications it causes can be very serious. Most severe pelvic infections occurred with a specific IUD that was taken off the market years ago, but if a pelvic infection does occur, it is much more serious when there is an IUD. The chances of this happening are much less in a monogamous relationship.

If a woman gets pregnant, her IUD must be removed. This can be very difficult to do in the office because the IUD can be drawn well into the pregnant uterus. If it can't be removed, some doctors advocate aborting since the IUD will cause severe infection, premature labor, and breaking the bag of water.

The birth control pill is the most popular contraceptive in the United States. It is the most effective, easy form to use, and it has some positive side effects. For example, it reduces menstrual flow and pain, may prevent PMS in some women, and makes cycles regular. It lowers the chances of getting uterine and ovarian cancer, ovarian cysts, and even pelvic inflammatory disease. It can decrease hair growth and acne in some women as well.

The standard pill keeps a steady, high level of estrogen and progesterone in the body, which tricks it into thinking it has already ovulated. It is considered low risk for women of all ages, although the risk of stroke and heart attack become significant for smokers when they reach thirty-five.

"The Pill" is actually taken as a series of oral tablets. It is started on the first day of the period, or on the first Sunday after the period starts, depending on the type of pill. The first twenty-one pills are hormonally active and prevent a woman from menstruating. The next seven pills are sugar pills. During that week, the body's estrogen and progesterone levels drop, just as in a natural menstrual cycle, and the uterine lining is shed in response.

During the first month or two that women take the Pill, it is normal to have nausea, bloating, and irregular bleeding. These symptoms usually stop by the third month. If one type of pill causes too many side effects, there are many others that can be tried. The Pill does not interfere with future fertility. A woman may try to get pregnant a month or two after stopping, although it may take a few months for her to get back into a regular cycle.

The estrogen in one type of pill reduces milk production, so nursing women take progesterone-only pills known as minipills, Micronor, or NorQD. These don't affect the baby and might even increase milk a bit. These don't always prevent ovulation, but they do interfere with fertilization and implantation. Since these pills need to be taken at exactly the same time every day, they are not used when the regular pill will do.

Progesterone shots are given every three months, and they cause weight gain and bleeding irregularities. Progesterone implants are placed in the arm every year. Their use is reserved for women who would otherwise not use contraception appropriately.

Tubal ligation is a way of sterilizing women where the woman's Fallopian tubes are tied off. Its main drawback is that women never know if life circumstances will one day be such that they will want to have more children.

Having Another Baby

Many women who want more than one child wonder how long their uterus needs to rest before they can optimally have another pregnancy.

Women who do not breastfeed often ovulate as soon as four weeks after giving birth. Women who breastfeed vary in how long it takes to resume ovulation, but the majority will ovulate by six months after delivery.

The *New England Journal of Medicine* recently published an article that looked at what happened to 173,000 pregnancies of women who already had three or more children. They found that pregnancies that were conceived less than six months after the prior birth had a greater chance of resulting in a low-birth-weight baby or one who was born prematurely. This may be because the mother's nutritional stores are depleted, and her body is not equipped for the physical and emotional stress of having two pregnancies and births so close together. When pregnancies were spaced eighteen to twenty-three months apart, the babies were born with the least amount of problems.

Page numbers in *italics* indicate illustrations; those in **bold** indicate tables.

Dr. Boris Petrikovsky is the chairman of obstetrics and gynecology at Nassau University Medical Center in East Meadow, New York, and a professor of obstetrics and gynecology at New York University School of Medicine. He has received awards and honors internationally for his research work. He has written over one hundred research articles in his twenty-five years as a specialist in maternal-fetal medicine. He is world renowned for his research and is a sought-after speaker throughout the world at conferences and medical conventions.

Dr. Jessica Jacob received a B.A. from New York University in Fine Arts, and her M.D. from New York University School of Medicine. She did her residency in obstetrics and gynecology at North Shore University Hospital before going into private practice, where she has delivered over three thousand babies. Dr. Jacob has been a guest on *The Today Show* and *The Phil Donahue Show,* and has been featured in *Working Mother* magazine and *New York Newsday.* She is the mother of seven children.

Dr. Lisa Aiken received her Ph.D. in clinical psychology at Loyola University of Chicago. She is the former chief psychologist of Lenox Hill Hospital and has a private psychotherapy practice with individuals and couples in New York City and Great Neck, New York. She has authored five books and lectures worldwide on a variety of topics. She is listed in twelve *Who's Who* directories and has appeared on radio and television.